Homoeopathy
FOR WOMEN

A Guide to Vital Health

Beth MacEoin

Headway · Hodder & Stoughton

The information in this book is advisory in nature and should not be regarded as a replacement for the services of a health professional. If in doubt, consult your GP or homoeopathic practitioner. Neither the publishers nor the author accept responsibility for the consequences of self-treatment.

A catalogue record for this title is available from the British Library

ISBN 0340 61892 2

First published 1995

| Impression number | 10 | 9 | 8 | 7 | 6 | 5 | 4 | 3 | 2 | 1 |
| Year | | 1999 | 1998 | 1997 | 1996 | 1995 | | | | |

Typeset by Wearset, Boldon, Tyne and Wear.
Printed in Great Britain for Hodder & Stoughton Educational, a division of Hodder Headline Plc, 338 Euston Road, London NW1 3BH by Cox & Wyman Ltd, Reading

CONTENTS

FOREWORD

Women, whatever their age, will be familiar with some of the health problems in this book. What many may not be familiar with is the concept of a holistic approach to good health, and the life-enhancing benefits this can bring. To realise there are things you can do for yourself, things which make a *real* difference, is exhilarating. Such an approach gives back responsibility to the woman as she realises there is often another choice, and she can share in deciding how she will develop that choice herself.

In easy-to-read terms Beth explains about homoeopathy, its history and basic philosophy, and gives a series of remedy snapshots in chart form for easy reference. Some of these pictures are explored in depth later in the book. She takes us through a number of common health conditions, and describes basic self-help measures, the homoeopathic approach, and the conventional approach. She makes clear the circumstances in which further help should be sought from a professionally qualified homoeopath, other alternative practitioner, or medical practitioner. She makes no judgements about which approach should be taken, but rather sets out to inform end empower.

Beth's enthusiasm for her subject is obvious, based on comprehensive training, experience in practice and the benefits she has seen at first hand. She is a committed professional homoeopath, keen to encourage her patients and

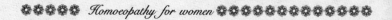

readers into thinking and acting positively about their health.

This book is one you can read, refer to, and return to time and time again.

Mary Clarke
General Secretary
The Society of Homoeopaths

ACKNOWLEDGEMENTS

Thanks are due to the following for their support and involvement with this project: Mary Clark, Sue Hart, Dr. Tessa Katz, Angela Morse, and Teresa Chris. My mother, Nancy, was, as always, an inspiration in the background. Special thanks are also due to my husband Denis for this unfailing critical judgement and extra-special editorial advice, without which I would be lost.

Beth MacEoin

For Denis, with all my love

INTRODUCTION

Increasingly large numbers of patients are being drawn towards homoeopathy as a system of alternative medicine, and it is striking that a very large proportion of these patients are women. Many of us will have become excited at the prospect of healing that homoeopathy provides, with its emphasis on the essential importance of treating the whole person and bringing our emotions, mind and body back into an optimum state of harmony and equilibrium. When this occurs, our perception of well-being is enhanced, our energy levels are increased, and we often feel as though we are at last fulfilling our creative potential.

This is because homoeopathy, in common with other holistic systems of healing, is not concerned with suppressing individual symptoms, but seeks to stimulate the body's own self-healing potential. As a result, our understanding of good health takes on a positive colouring, as something far more exciting and profound than the mere absence of disease or troublesome symptoms.

Taking on a radical holistic perspective, we soon start to see that there are practical steps we can take to achieve and maintain an improved experience of positive good health. Once we begin to move along this path the exhilaration that follows can be immense, as we appreciate that we can take far more responsibility for improving the quality of our health than we may have previously considered possible.

The information contained in this book is designed to

help you take the first step along this journey. In it you will find a range of common complaints, with advice on how to approach each problem from the perspective of prevention, together with general self-help measures, including exercise, relaxation, and dietary adjustments. In the treatment tables you will find a run-down of appropriate homoeopathic medicines, plus advice on conditions that may be treated with self-prescribing, as well as those that should be treated by a trained practitioner.

Although a little daunting and challenging at first, learning how to use homoeopathic medicines at home can be an immensely fulfilling and empowering experience. I wish you successful and rewarding prescribing.

CHAPTER 1

HOMOEOPATHY: THE BASICS

Women and homoeopathy

Women have been directly involved with the history of homoeopathy from a very early stage. The first woman to practise as a homoeopathic physician was Melanie Hahnemann, the second wife of Samuel Hahnemann, the founder of modern homoeopathic medicine. A remarkably emancipated woman for her time, Melanie was also a key influence in the busy Paris practice of her husband.

This tradition continues today, with the majority of homoeopathic practitioners, teachers, and students being women. Homoeopaths also see very large numbers of female patients who seek treatment for a range of conditions including health problems that are commonly seen as part of being a woman. These include painful or irregular periods, pre-menstrual syndrome (PMS), cystitis, hot flushes and other menopausal problems.

One of the reasons why homoeopathy is particularly attractive to women may be the fact that they play the role of carers on a day-to-day basis. If a member of the family falls ill, or if an elderly relative needs looking after, care is usually provided by the wife, mother or daughter, depending on the individual situation. Within a hospital context, nurses are

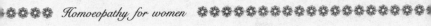

predominantly female, while community care is provided by women in the form of health visitors, community nurses and midwives.

From this perspective it is hardly surprising that women play a vital role in the practice of holistic forms of healing such as homoeopathy, with their emphasis on the need for empathy, understanding, and caring for the individual as a whole person on mental, emotional and physical levels.

What is homoeopathy?

Homoeopathy is a system of healing that has been in existence for roughly 200 years. It is practised worldwide by both conventional doctors and professional homoeopaths. In trained hands, it provides a method of restoring the unwell person to optimum health in a gentle, effective, thorough and balanced way.

The concept of similars

The word 'homoeopathy' comes from a Greek source, and roughly translated means 'similar suffering'. In other words, the substance that triggers disease in a healthy person can be used as a healing agent when given to a sick person, provided her symptoms resemble those of the agent. The concept of using similar medicines dates at least from the time of the ancient Greek physician Hippocrates, but Samuel Hahnemann, the originator of homoeopathy as a coherent medical system, developed the basic concept into a complete therapeutic system with an elaborate philosophical basis. In doing so, he established an extremely controversial theory of health and disease that went completely against the grain of the current medical thinking of his day. This conflict continues to this day, with some orthodox scientists regarding homoeopathic theories of healing as contradicting and falling outside the basic premises of scientific thinking.

Instead of counteracting the symptoms of illness by suppression, Hahnemann recommended the use of medicines that supported the body's self-healing mechanism. He regarded the symptoms of disease as an expression of the body's own fruitless attempt to throw off internal stresses and toxins. From this perspective, Hahnemann developed a theory of healing that was more concerned with stimulating the body's defence mechanism than weakening it through violent measures such as bleeding and purging, or the use of arsenic, mercury and other toxic substances in large quantities. These drastic measures with their terrible consequences were very fashionable in the conventional medical circles of Hahnemann's day.

Provings of remedies

Hahnemann carried out a series of controlled experiments on himself and other volunteers in order to find out what effects a medicinal substance would have on a healthy individual. He called these experiments 'provings'. They involved taking small amounts of a substance repeatedly and recording the effects in minute detail. The people selected were in good health at the time of the experiment, and ready to observe and record any changes in their emotional or physical health for as long as the experiment continued. Today many hundreds of homoeopathic medicines are in use which have been proved in this way, and the process continues to develop as new medicines are introduced.

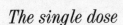

The single dose

Since the original provings were carried out using single substances rather than compounds, homoeopathic medicines are commonly given as single remedies. Reactions are noted, and the decision is made whether to wait, repeat, move on to a different strength, or change the remedy altogether.

One of the strongest arguments in favour of the administration of one remedy at a time is that it is very difficult to assess how effective a particular remedy has been if it is closely followed by, or mixed with, another. Because of the tradition of proving single substances rather than compounds or mixtures, detailed information on medicinal effects of the latter is not available.

The minimum dose

As well as the concept of using similar agents, Hahnemann also developed the idea that the dose of the medicine administered should be the smallest amount possible to stimulate self-healing. This preoccupation of his can be traced back to the appalling side-effects from drugs that he witnessed during his career as an orthodox doctor. He was, therefore, motivated to experiment using increasingly smaller doses of medicines until he came to a point where orthodox medical science parted company with him. Although no molecules of the original substance could be traced at this level of dilution, Hahnemann discovered that these highly dilute medicines had a profound effect in stimulating the self-healing properties of the body, provided they were subjected to an additional process of 'succussion', or vigorous shaking, at each stage of dilution.

As long as the essential similarity between the symptoms of the patient and the medicine existed, Hahnemann discovered that the more dilute a homoeopathic remedy became, the stronger the curative effect proved to be – always provided it had gone through succussion at each stage of dilution.

Homoeopathy treats people, not diseases

The concept of treating each person as an individual who responds to illness in her own way is central to homoeopathic practice. Any changes or disturbances that have appeared on physical, mental or emotional levels since the illness began must be paid attention to: it is an analysis of this vital information which will lead the practitioner to choose the most appropriate homoeopathic medicine.

Although a basic label can be given to a group of common symptoms in order to provide a diagnosis, no two people experience illness in quite the same way. If we take the basic example of two women suffering from flu, both might have the general symptoms of fever, aching, lack of energy, sore throat, runny nose, and cough. However, this general information will not help the homoeopath in searching for the appropriate prescription, since it tells nothing about the way each individual is expressing her illness.

In order to discover this, it is necessary to probe more deeply into the individual characteristics of each woman's symptoms to see a sharper picture emerging. Once we begin to observe and question more closely, we discover that one woman fell ill rapidly within a matter of hours and soon developed a high temperature. Since falling ill, all she wanted to do was sit in a quiet, dark room to try to relieve the severe headache that came on with the fever. Any

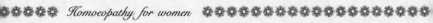

disturbance or stimulation from well-meaning family or friends would make her feel worse. Although very sleepy and drowsy, she couldn't get to sleep from the pain in her head and severe sore throat. Trying to drink made the throat worse, and even though her mouth was dry she was not thirsty. Her skin was dry, bright red, and so hot that it radiated heat. Although feeling so hot, the patient complained of terrific cold-sensitivity and aggravation of symptoms from contact with the least draught of cold air.

The other woman began to feel ill slowly, being aware of a sore throat that got progressively worse as the day went on. Her symptoms were much worse at night, when she became unusually anxious and restless. Normally calm by nature with no problems getting to sleep, she was very anxious and distressed about being alone at night. Although her throat was sore and burning, sipping warm drinks made her throat much more comfortable. She also complained of unusual chilliness, and felt much better for being in bed with a hot-water bottle. Although feverish at night, she looked pale and drawn rather than flushed.

In these two simple examples we can see straight away how each woman is expressing her symptoms in her own individual way. It would be of no help to give them both the same homoeopathic medicine, since their specific symptoms are different (even though they share general features of the illness). Unless an exact match exists between the symptoms of a sick person and the features of a homoeopathic remedy, no amount of an inappropriately chosen medicine will be of help in stimulating cure. In this case, the first woman needed Belladonna, and the second Arsenicum album. This is because a sick person is being prescribed for, not an abstract disease label.

Homoeopathy and orthodox medicine

In order to grasp fully the marked contrast between homoeopathic and orthodox views of health and disease with particular regard to the treatment of women's health problems, we first need to explore the context in which Samuel Hahnemann developed his original ideas.

Homoeopathy: The early days

Samuel Hahnemann was born in 1755 in Meissen, Germany and qualified as a doctor in 1779. The more he witnessed of fashionable orthodox medical procedures such as bleeding (through leeching and cupping), purging by using vast quantities of drastic laxatives, and the use of highly poisonous substances such as mercury to treat venereal disease, the more convinced he became that he was doing more harm than good by practising as an orthodox doctor.

As a result he made the decision to stop practising as a physician in 1796 and put his efforts into translating foreign medical texts. He was also motivated to conduct his own experiments into more gentle and less barbaric ways of treating patients than he had observed during his time as an orthodox doctor.

While he was translating Cullen's *Materia Medica*, Hahnemann was intrigued and puzzled by the author's explanation for the effectiveness of cinchona bark as a successful medical substance in treating the symptoms of malaria. Cullen's explanation that it was the astringent properties of cinchona bark that rendered it medicinally effective did not satisfy Hahnemann, who decided to conduct his own experiments in order to see if another explanation presented itself. As a result, Hahnemann took repeated doses

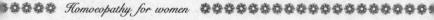

of cinchona bark himself, and observed and recorded its effects. He found that while he continued the dosage, he began to develop malaria symptoms which went away once he stopped taking the medicine. As a direct result of this experience, he began the long and tortuous path of developing the theory and practice of homoeopathy: the treatment of sick individuals with similar substances rather than opposites. He continually developed and updated his ideas in the search for the gentlest way of restoring sick people to good health, until his death in Paris in 1843.

After working further along these lines, expanding the range of medicines used, Hahnemann began to pay attention to the problem of how to lessen any adverse side-effects that the medicines caused. He began to use increasingly smaller and more dilute doses of medicine in an effort to produce the gentlest and most humane form of treatment. Then came a vital point where he made a quantum leap in his thinking by adding the systematic repetition of vigorous pounding or 'succussion' at each stage of dilution. He found that these two procedures had to be carried out in order for a medicine to be prepared homoeopathically. This process came to be called 'potentization'.

The more he observed of these potentized medicines, the more he discovered that the reactions he observed ran against the grain of anything that could be explained by the scientific discoveries and theories of his day. He discovered that the more dilute and succussed a medicine became (even to the point where there was no remaining molecule of the original substance present), the more powerful the effect appeared to be on the sick person, provided the essential 'similarity' of the patient's symptom picture as a whole matched that of the prescribed remedy.

The next step: Developing the concept of vital energy

As Hahnemann developed and refined his ideas, he came to the conclusion that there must be some basic intelligence which regulated the harmonious functioning of the human body as a whole and preserved a fluid but balanced state of health. When this basic intelligence or 'vital force' came in contact with a stressful stimulus which it could not resist, symptoms of illness or dis-ease would develop. These symptoms would be a sign of the body's own dynamic but ineffective attempt to achieve self-healing, giving clues as to the nature of the imbalance, and also providing vital information for the selection of the appropriate homoeopathic medicine.

If we take this approach, we begin to see symptoms of illness in a much more positive light than we would from an orthodox medical perspective.

Health, disease and orthodox medicine

Conventional medicine regards the human body as constantly under siege from hostile invaders, such as bacteria and viruses. As a result, medical research works along the lines of searching for the 'magic bullet' which will fight and destroy the invader. In contrast with homoeopathy, which aims to stimulate and support the body's own self-healing potential to overcome infection, orthodox medicine works by identifying the harmful organism through investigations and tests in order to deal with it by giving the appropriate drug.

Orthodox drugs are also very different in preparation and prescription when compared with the way homoeopathic medicines are prepared and selected. Because homoeopathic medicines are understood to work by stimulating our body's self-defence mechanism, they support and enable it to fight disease more efficiently. Orthodox or 'allopathic' drugs, however, work in quite a different way, since they are selected on the basis of their counteracting disease symptoms by producing an opposite effect. Familiar examples of this process include the use of antacids to counter over-acidity in the stomach, laxatives for constipation, antibiotics to eliminate bacteria, and anti-inflammatories to dampen down inflammation. Because these drugs work by counteracting symptoms, they often need to be repeated at regular intervals or take on a long-term basis in order to keep symptoms under control.

The homoeopathic approach is quite different since it concentrates on supporting and encouraging the body to work more efficiently so that it can come to terms with, and overcome, symptoms itself. As a result, the long-term aim of successful homoeopathic treatment is to get the body in a sufficient degree of balance so that further intervention is unnecessary unless, and until, the body is again overwhelmed by stress.

Limitations of conventional medicine

One of the main drawbacks and limitations of orthodox medical treatment is the preoccupation with common disease symptoms in pursuit of the appropriate drug therapy. As a result, it is easy to lose sight of the individual while pursuing the correct diagnosis. This often has the unhappy result of leaving us feeling as though we are little more than

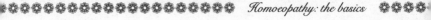

a walking disease label: a feeling which is often unknowingly reinforced by the range of investigative procedures and tests to which we are exposed in pursuit of diagnosis and treatment.

Because conventional medicine perceives good health as the absence of disease, rather than the positive acquisition of a healthy and well-balanced body, we often are led to expect a pill to deal with every minor problem that may surface with regard to our health. This is often the result of doctors losing sight of our bodies as integrated systems that possess a defence mechanism of their own, which, when healthy and in good working order, can fight off illness decisively and effectively. As a result, many of us have lost touch with the basic knowledge we can use to help ourselves or our families through straightforward and short-term infections, such as the common cold.

Sensible supportive measures such as increasing fluid intake, keeping food light and easily digestible, resting as much as possible, and avoiding extreme changes of temperature while feverish, will all be helpful in aiding our bodies to fight infection more effectively. Unfortunately, many of us are tempted to take pills to mask unpleasant symptoms temporarily in an effort to keep going, only to discover that we take longer to recover, with an added risk of developing complications such as a chest infection or repeated relapses. This is the legacy of the magic bullet, which unwittingly encourages us to ignore or suppress the important signals our body is sending us that we may need to take it easy for a few days in order to recover fully.

When homoeopathy is used appropriately and effectively, it supports us through the stages of illness speedily and with the minimum risk of complications. If we take the common cold as an example, competent homoeopathic prescribing is unlikely to stop the illness in its tracks, but it can speed up the progress of cure and make the risk of extended chest or sinus problems less likely. Because homoeopathy works by assisting the body in its attempt to resolve disease, any measures that assist the body in this fight will be supportive of homoeopathic treatment. This is why a large proportion of this book is devoted to basic self-help measures and general advice about maintaining optimum health, as well as basic information regarding homoeopathic remedies for each condition.

The advantages of a holistic approach towards healing for women

Women in particular have tended to suffer from problem areas of their bodies being 'compartmentalised' so that they can be dealt with in manageable chunks. In other words, if we have problems with our periods we may be treated by a gynaecologist, if we are experiencing long-term, or severe emotional trauma we will see a psychotherapist, or if the problem seems to be hormonal, we may be sent to an endocrinologist. By the time we have been through this process, it is hardly surprising that we begin to see ourselves as a series of unrelated parts, all requiring treatment in isolation from each other.

In contrast to this approach, homoeopathic medicine has at its heart the concept of the vital importance of treating the whole person rather than a series of parts in isolation. From this positive perspective, links are stressed between the mind and body, and between imbalances in general health and emotional well-being. This emphasis on the ultimate

need to create harmony between mind and body in order to enjoy health at its most positive level makes homoeopathy a particularly positive and beneficial therapy for those of us who have felt unsatisfied with the conventional medical approach. This is not to suggest that men cannot and do not frequently benefit from homoeopathy as a therapy; it is, rather, a way of highlighting the special potential that homoeopathy provides for women who are unhappy or uneasy about their problems being treated in isolation without the consequences for their sense of well-being as a whole being considered.

Homoeopathy as a way of achieving essential harmony and balance between mind and body

The stresses and pressures on women are enormous: all too often we have to juggle pursuing a career, running a home and caring for a family, with the expectation that we will feel clear-headed and energised at the end of a working day. The 'superwoman' myth has a lot to answer for, since its unfortunate victims often end in grief, with many of them feeling overburdened, stressed, exhausted, sick, and not surprisingly, often resentful.

If we turn to conventional medicine we may be offered a drug to calm us down, to help us sleep, or even to iron out our moods so that we experience no 'highs' or 'lows' any more. While they may offer temporary help and support, it is in the nature of these drugs that they may lead to addiction, fatigue, and lack of dynamism and vitality.

The other possible scenario is that problems may become

centred on a specific group of symptoms, such as pre-
menstrual tension, so that we experience severe mood swings
including irritability and depression and a host of physical
symptoms as well, such as fluid retention, breast tenderness,
and severely painful periods. If we seek conventional
treatment we may be given diuretics to help deal with fluid
retention, or painkillers to ease the pain, but once again, the
whole person is being lost somewhere in the middle of these
separate compartments. In other words, the orthodox
medical approach is not designed to take the whole picture
into account, nor is it likely to help the individual woman
make the necessary connections to see what is happening to
her as an individual, so the root of the problem often goes
untreated, leaving the patient feeling lost and helpless. In
this situation, the crucial balance between mind and body
has usually been lost sight of, which only leads to increased
feelings of confusion and fear.

On the other hand, homoeopathy is a system of healing
that emphasises the need for stimulation of a sense of well-
being on emotional and physical levels if we are to
experience optimum health. Because homoeopathy is
essentially an energy-based system of medicine, stimulating
energy potential is the first step to dealing with health
problems. Once energy levels begin to improve, a sense of
well-being may be established and physical symptoms recede
into the background. From the perspective of the
'fragmented' woman, we can see that this is a system of
health care which has obvious advantages, stressing as it does
the need to get the whole person into balance.

CHAPTER 2

HOMOEOPATHY IN ACTION: HOW TO USE THIS BOOK

Conditions which are appropriate for home prescribing

You will find a range of conditions listed in the following chapters, some of which will respond effectively and decisively to self-help measures and short-term homoeopathic prescribing. These include the occasional headache, bout of indigestion, or attack of cystitis that comes out of the blue. These are conditions that we can regard as **acute**; in other words, they are short-lived, and will often clear up of their own accord given appropriate supportive help from basic measures such as rest and dietary improvements.

- However, there are other conditions listed in this book for which it is essential to seek professional advice. These include pre-menstrual syndrome, endometriosis, ME (chronic fatigue syndrome), arthritis and acne. Generally speaking, these are problems that are subject to repeated flare-ups over an extended period of time, and do not rectify themselves, no matter how much time goes by. This category of health problem can be identified as a **chronic** condition.

It is also important to stress that the conditions mentioned above, such as headaches, cystitis and indigestion, can also turn into a chronic problem if they occur at frequent intervals. If this is the case, it is important to seek professional help rather than attempting to deal with the situation yourself. On the other hand, if you do not normally suffer headaches or indigestion, but experience either after an unusual bout of overindulgence, this would fall into the acute category and it is appropriate to try home prescribing as well as other self-help measures.

You will also find that some of the chronic conditions listed in this book have homoeopathic remedy tables included, even though it is not recommended that you attempt self-prescribing. This is done in order to show the scope of treatment that will be available from a professional source, and to stress that it is not uncommon for homoeopaths to treat patients who suffer from such a condition. In some situations, it is recommended that you initially try general self-help measures to see if these help your condition substantially (this may or may not include short-term use of an appropriate homoeopathic medicine). If your condition does not improve within a reasonable time, the suggestion will be made that you need to seek professional help and advice.

It is necessary to seek professional help when dealing with chronic problems because case management can be complicated, and the training and expertise of a professional is needed in order to guide the patient towards a general state of improved health. This is especially true where a skin condition such as eczema or acne is involved, since homoeopaths generally view a long-term skin eruption as indicative of a deep-seated, often inherited, disorder which needs to be dealt with before the whole person can enjoy improved health. If the skin condition is combined with a more internal disorder, such as hay fever or asthma, very skilful case management is needed to achieve overall improvement of the case. In situations such as these, the homoeopath must constantly use his or her professional judgement and experience to assess how the patient is progressing.

This is because homoeopathy is a system of healing which is not concerned with haphazard suppression or removal of symptoms, but is attempting to restore the sick individual to health in the most profound sense. When this happens, symptoms improve as good health is established on mental, emotional and physical levels. For this reason, there are certain guidelines that can be used by homoeopathic practitioners to establish that a case is moving in a curative direction. These involve the following:

- **Symptoms improve in reverse order of their appearance**. In other words, the most recent symptom to appear is the first to improve, and the most established is the last to leave.

- **Symptoms improve from within outwards**. Therefore, we anticipate that a condition centring on more internal organs (digestive problems, such as heartburn, or respiratory symptoms, such as bronchitis or asthma) will improve before a skin condition, such as psoriasis.

- **Symptoms move in a downward direction**. For example, if someone is suffering from eczema, eruptions will often improve initially on the face and neck, moving down over chest, arms, hands and legs, until the condition has cleared up. This is also true of joint pains or muscle aches, which can improve in the upper body before leaving the lower limbs.

A note of caution

Care should be taken with any of the conditions listed in this book as suitable for home prescribing if they show any signs of increasing in severity, or if you suspect serious complications are developing. You will find suggestions at the end of each section which indicate that professional help is needed. Within this context, such help should come from your GP, or in rare situations where time is short, the emergency department of your nearest hospital. In less urgent situations, existing patients of a professional or doctor homoeopath should notify their practitioner of the situation. If you do not have immediate access to a homoeopathic practitioner, you can contact your GP initially, and after the immediate situation has been dealt with, consider finding a homoeopathic practitioner to investigate the problem more deeply. For information about finding a suitable practitioner, see the section in Chapter 7, entitled How do I find a homoeopathic practitioner? (page 171).

It is also worth pointing out that if you are consulting a homoeopath, it is unwise to continue with self-help for acute problems without informing your practitioner. It is likely that they will deal with any acute prescriptions that you may need, and that they will check these are compatible with your 'constitutional' treatment. The latter is aimed at dealing with your individual underlying predisposition to illness.

Always follow your instinct if you suspect you may be getting out of your depth, and never be reluctant to ask for professional help if you suspect a condition could be serious: in this situation it is always most prudent to err on the side of caution.

Using this book: Selecting the right remedy

In order to obtain the best results when using this book, you should do the following:

• Using a note pad and pencil, write down any symptoms you have noticed since the illness began. This refers as much to subjective changes, such as emotional disturbances, as well as easily observable symptoms, such as paleness in a person who normally has a rosy complexion.

• Bear in mind that you are only interested in changes from the normal healthy state of the sick person. In other words, if someone is normally chilly, you would not attach importance to this. However, if the same person complains of feeling hot and flushed since feeling ill, this would be a valid symptom, because it signifies a change from their normal state.

• Once you have completed your list, isolate any symptoms that you regard as being peculiar or unusual. For instance, chilliness with aversion to heat, burning pains that feel better for warmth, or nausea that is relieved by eating. These are vital symptoms that may be invaluable in clinching your choice of remedy.

• Look for a characteristic or theme running through the symptoms. For example, dryness may be a common characteristic running through sensations in the throat, bowel movements, and skin texture. If you have a unifying thread like this running through the symptoms, they cease to be a jumbled list of random

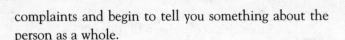

complaints and begin to tell you something about the person as a whole.

• Take into account any precipitating factors which may have been present before illness set in, such as becoming chilled, or several nights' disturbed sleep, or severe emotional strain, shock or fright. This is always worth noting.

• Find out what makes the patient feel generally better or worse. This may apply to factors which improve or aggravate specific symptoms, or which have a more general effect on the person as a whole.

• Always pay attention to and note any changes which have occurred on an emotional level since illness set in. Weepiness in a normally cheery person, or anxiety and restlessness in a normally relaxed individual, are always symptoms of value.

• By now you should have a fairly long list of symptoms which you can divide into headings such as **causative factors, general symptoms** and **modalities** (things which make the patient feel better or worse).

• Bear in mind that the general symptom heading can cover a wide scope, referring to any changes from normal on both emotional and physical levels.

• Turn to the appropriate table in the relevant section of the book. Look down the left-hand column entitled *Type* to see which category fits the group of symptoms you have on paper most closely. If you have identified a causative factor, this will help you a great deal at this point. This column will also give you information about what stage of illness you may be thinking of, in other words, whether it refers to early onset, or a more established stage of illness.

• Once you have found the category you want, check the information under the heading *General indications* and see how it matches the general symptoms you have noted. Don't worry unduly if you can't find all the symptoms you have noted under that heading, since it is extremely unlikely that you will ever find a perfect match between the two. What you must assess is whether the most central features of the general indications match with the symptoms you regard as important. For example, you would consider Pulsatilla as a strong candidate if the patient is chilly, but much better for cool air and gentle exercise, and worse for heat and resting, weepy, and craving company and sympathy. If, however, the patient feels much worse for crying, any physical expression of sympathy and comfort from others, and much better when left by themselves, we need to look at another remedy such as Natrum mur to find a close match between general symptoms and the appropriate homoeopathic remedy.

• If you are unsure about what symptoms represent the major central features of a homoeopathic medicine, consult the section at the back of the book entitled **Keynotes**. This will give you a quick overview of the essential features running through each remedy.

• If you feel satisfied that the match between the symptom you have listed and the homoeopathic medicine you are considering is close enough, look at the columns entitled *Worse from* and *Better for*. If these

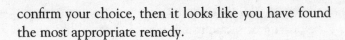

confirm your choice, then it looks like you have found the most appropriate remedy.

• Remember, what you are looking for is the information which characterises what is individual in the sick person's symptoms. Always search for what it is that makes one individual's case of cystitis or indigestion different from another's. Common symptoms such as fever, headache, or restlessness will not help you at all in your search for the appropriate homoeopathic remedy. You must always try to discover how these broad symptoms affect the individual in the way they experience pain, fever, or anxiety, and how these symptoms affect their systems as a whole.

• You will soon observe that certain medicines appear under different sections. For instance Arsenicum album appears in the tables for short-term insomnia, ME, and 'empty nest' syndrome, while Pulsatilla appears in the tables for hot flushes, acne, and morning sickness. By familiarising yourself with these tables and the Keynotes at the back of the book, you will begin to grasp the idea of these being multi-faceted medicines that cover a broad range of health problems in their own individual way. As you become more familiar with their use you will begin to discover how each remedy has its own individual characteristics, just as the woman who is unwell manifests her illness in a way that is unique to her. Although you may initially feel confused or overwhelmed by the scope of each remedy picture, don't worry unduly. As you use the medicines on a regular basis for short-lived problems, each one will become familiar to you.

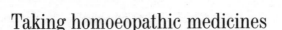

Taking homoeopathic medicines

Homoeopathic medicines are usually given in tablet form, but they can also be administered as globules, granules, liquids, and powders, or applied to the skin as diluted tinctures, creams or ointments.

• Tip out a single dose of your selected remedy (a single dose being one tablet) onto a clean spoon.

• Do not wash the tablet down with a drink, but suck or chew it in a clean mouth. Remember that a clean mouth does not mean that you need to brush your teeth before taking a remedy, but refers to the fact that you should avoid eating, drinking or brushing your teeth too close to taking the remedy. It's a good idea to leave a margin of half an hour either side of eating or drinking.

• Homoeopaths often suggest that you should avoid the use of strong tea, coffee, peppermint, or the application of strong-smelling camphor rubs or aromatic oils. These also include essential oils commonly used in aromatherapy such as peppermint, rosemary, eucalyptus and thyme. It is generally a good idea to avoid any of these substances where possible, especially if you are new to homoeopathic prescribing. By removing these factors from the equation, you avoid any potential confusion if it looks as though the remedy you have selected is not working.

• Store your remedies away from strong odours, bright light, or extreme variations of temperature. A fairly cool, dark place is usually most suitable (but not

as cool as your fridge). If your remedies are stored under
these conditions they will remain medicinally active for
years, since they are well-known as having a very long
'shelf life'.

• If you accidentally spill some tablets out of the
bottle, do not put them back in, throw them away.

Repeating the remedy

• Take the first dose of your indicated remedy as
suggested in the previous section. Wait for half an hour;
if you observe no change, repeat the same remedy. You
can repeat the same dose up to three times at intervals
of half an hour.

• Once you observe the first signs of any change in
the condition, **stop** taking the remedy. This is an
indication that the body is now doing the work for
itself, and that continuing the remedy will be unnecessary unless, and until, the symptoms return. Once
again, as soon as you observe an improvement, stop
taking the remedy.

• The repetition suggested above is the recommended dose for a condition of sudden and recent onset,
such as a bout of cystitis, thrush, or headache. However, if your condition has been building up gradually
over a number of days, or if it is more well established,
you are likely to respond more favourably to repetition
of the appropriate remedy three or four times daily over
a period of three to four days. As before, as soon as you
observe any marked change in your condition, **stop**
taking the remedy. If an improvement is gaining

momentum, you do not need another dose of the remedy unless a relapse occurs.

• If you do not experience an improvement within the suggested time, take another look at the appropriate table and consider if another remedy may be more suitable. You will also need to do this if your symptoms have changed since taking the remedy you first selected, in order to find a closer match to the modified symptoms. If one remedy hasn't worked, there is no problem of incompatibility in moving to another which may be more effective. Because the medicines work at a sub-molecular level, there is no risk of any chemical residue being left in the body which might spark off a toxic reaction.

• You will find that most health food shops and high street chemists stock a reasonable range of homoeopathic medicines, usually in the 6c strength, and occasionally in 30c (See page 28). If the condition you are prescribing for is fairly mild and of recent onset (within the last hour or two), it is best initially to use the 6c potency, and only move on to the 30c if improvement is sluggish or very partial. It is better to begin with a 12c (available by telephone order from one of the homoeopathic pharmacies listed at the back of the book) or 30c if the condition has been longer established and the symptoms are more severe.

• It cannot be stressed enough that homoeopathic medicines are **not** designed to be taken over an extended period of time for acute (short-lived) or chronic (long-term) disorders. If you feel you need to take them on a daily basis to achieve and maintain an

improvement, it is essential that you seek more deep-seated 'constitutional' help from a homoeopathic practitioner.

• Above all else, if you are feeling confused, unsure of what to do next, or generally out of your depth, always **seek professional help**. For a definition of 'professional help' please see page 18.

Do remember that it is the potency and frequency of repetition of the remedy that determines the length and strength of its action, rather than the size of the dose. In other words, if you took one, two, or five tablets at the same time it would still count as a single dose of the remedy. However, if you took one tablet every ten minutes for an hour, this would count as six doses, since the remedy is being administered at regular intervals.

Which remedies should I buy?

It is very difficult to be specific about the exact selection needed in the average basic self-help kit, since one person's needs will not be the same as another's. For instance, the remedies included in a kit to meet the needs of a family including babies and young children will differ from those often indicated for a couple or a single person without children.

However, the following list of remedies will provide a good starter kit for someone prescribing for the majority of conditions discussed in this book, and also gives a sound foundation from which to develop a more broadly based selection of remedies.

Aconite	*Ignatia*
Arnica	*Lachesis*
Arsenicum album	*Natrum mur*
Belladonna	*Nux vomica*
Bryonia	*Pulsatilla*
Calc carb	*Sepia*
Gelsemium	

Useful additions would include the following:

Apis	*Mercurius*
Carbo veg	*Phosphorus*
Ipecac	*Rhus tox*
Hepar sulph	*Staphysagria*
Lycopodium	*Sulphur*

The following creams and tinctures are also invaluable:

Calendula or **Hypercal tincture** (a mixture of Calendula and Hypericum) to be used diluted on cuts, abrasions, or added to the bathwater after surgery or childbirth.

Calendula cream to be applied after Hypercal tincture in order to minimise the risk of infection, slow down bleeding, and encourage speedy healing. Calendula ointment is also available for use on roughened or grazed skin that requires move intensive moisturizing.

These are, of course, arbitrary lists and should in no way be considered exhaustive or inflexible. There are many more 'basic' homoeopathic medicines, all of them useful, but the above should provide the beginner with a sound basis on which to build.

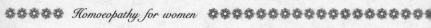

What potency should I buy?

Once again, this is a rather tricky question to answer, since different situations often require differing potencies of the appropriate homoeopathic medicine. For an explanation of potencies and their range of of usefulness please see the section entitled 'What does the word 'potency' refer to?' below. Generally speaking it is best to buy your remedies in the 6c potency, and supplement these with the same remedies in 12c and 30c later. Do not be unduly anxious about selecting the optimum potency in the early days: if you have selected the appropriate homoeopathic medicine, use either a 6c, 12c, or 30c, remembering that you will repeat 12c and 30c less frequently than a lower potency such as 6c.

What does the word 'potency' refer to?

You will discover that most of the homoeopathic medicines available to you in pharmacies and health food stores usually come in a 6c potency, or sometimes in 30c. The letter 'c' refers to the method of dilution that has been used (in this case the centesimal scale of dilution). This means that the original substance been rendered solvent and diluted in an alcohol solution. One drop of this is added to ninety-nine drops of distilled water or alcohol and shaken or 'succussed' to render the first potency or 1c. This process is repeated at each stage, taking one drop of the last potency and adding it to ninety-nine drops of dilutant.

You can also find remedies that have a d or x after the number which means that these have been diluted according to the decimal scale. This involves the same broad process that has been outlined above, but in this case the proportions used are one drop of dilutant to nine drops of alcohol or distilled water.

Where can I buy homoeopathic medicines?

You will find that there are increasingly large outlets for the sale of homoeopathic medicines which have grown proportionally in order to meet the demand for treatment. Many high street chemists now have basic stocks of homoeopathic medicines, and health food shops will also provide a decent choice.

An even more satisfactory source as regards the availability and choice of different potencies is provided by the number of homoeopathic pharmacies that manufacture and sell remedies. These have the added advantage of employing trained staff who can often answer basic questions relating to elementary homoeopathic prescribing, or who know where best to refer you for more detailed help and advice. These are also the best outlets to approach if you want to obtain a homoeopathic self-help kit: they often have a selection of their own, or will be happy to put one together of your own choice. If you do not have a local homoeopathic pharmacy (see the Useful Addresses section), you can usually place orders by telephone or in writing.

You can obtain homoeopathic medicines in the form of small or large tablets, granules, powders, pilules or in liquid form. Creams, ointments, lotions and tinctures are also available for external use.

How can I learn more about homoeopathic self-help?

If you enjoy using this book you will benefit greatly from attending one of the many classes on homoeopathic self-help or first-aid that are regularly held across the country. Although a book can provide you with the basic information about home prescribing, it inevitably cannot answer all the questions in the reader's mind. Once you have become familiar with this book, attending a homoeopathic first-aid class will provide you with the opportunity to discuss issues with other beginners, and your queries can be answered straight away by the practitioner who is running the class.

If you would like to obtain further information about self-help classes in your area it will be necessary to contact your local education authority (extra-mural studies), library, local Homoeopathic Group, or Homoeopathic College.

THE EARLY STAGE: TEENAGE PROBLEMS

The teenage years are often a phase of life we associate with emotional trauma, self-consciousness, and a host of problems associated with the turbulence of major hormonal changes. However, they are also the years when the potential for creativity, energy and vivacity can be higher than at any other time of our lives.

Holistic approaches such as homoeopathy, acupuncture, herbalism, and other alternative methods of healing can be invaluable in helping to release this potential creativity by bringing the mind and body into the optimum state of balance. Most of these therapies will also stress the role that changes in lifestyle can play in improving overall health and well-being on mental, emotional and physical levels.

In this chapter you will find a selection of conditions that often mar the positive enjoyment of this time of life. Some of them are suitable for homoeopathic self-prescribing, while others need professional help and advice. In addition, this chapter contains a wealth of general advice with regard to basic dietary, relaxation and exercise approaches that can contribute to positive changes.

For advice on how to use the remedy tables, please see the section entitled **Using this book: Selecting the right remedy** on page 19. To obtain the best results it is essential to read this information first and follow the directions as closely as possible, rather than attempting to use the tables without instructions.

Eating Disorders

P roblems in relation to food and eating patterns can affect us at any time in our lives. However, eating disorders tend to be a particularly common problem for young women in their teens, especially during or following puberty. For many young women, controlling their weight and intake of food is the only way they feel they can exercise control over the changes that are taking place in their bodies. Severely restricting the amount of food we eat has the effect of retarding or reversing the changes that take place during puberty. As a result, our periods will stop, or their onset will be delayed, breast size will diminish, and our bodies take on the angular appearance that is characteristic of the pre-pubescent state.

Eating disorders can be sparked off by emotional trauma, a growing sense of low self-esteem or lack of confidence, fear of sexuality, or a desire to escape the responsibilities of leaving childhood behind; or they can be an unconscious way of seeking an increased amount of care and attention.

Symptoms may include:

- An obsessive relationship with food. This often involves a preoccupation with certain foods that are forbidden because of their calorific content. These are the 'comfort' foods such as chocolate, puddings, chips, cakes, crisps and ice-cream. In other words, most of the foods that will have been given as rewards, or withheld as punishments, when we were small children.

- A constant preoccupation with the calorific value of food and a constant struggle to stay within a rigid limit. If we go outside this limit, the result is usually profound guilt.

- Frequent monitoring of weight, usually on a daily basis, or often three or four times in one day.

- A dissatisfaction with each goal that is reached as an 'ideal' weight. Where an eating disorder has been well established, this weight can never be reached since the goalposts are constantly moved: usually downwards to a lighter weight each time the initial desired weight loss has been achieved.

- Severe fluctuations in weight gain or loss, often swinging from one extreme to another through 'yo-yo' dieting.

- Reliance on laxatives or vomiting after eating in an effort to avoid weight gain. Anyone who has suffered from bulimia will be familiar with the cycle of bingeing, followed by vomiting and/or purging through laxatives until the next bout of bingeing begins.

- Eating disorders often go hand in hand with a tendency to exercise in an obsessive way, with great distress resulting from disruption of a regular exercise routine. In other words, exercising can be another method used to 'burn off' extra calories in an effort to maintain a low weight, or to control weight gain.

- Possible symptoms of eating disorders include irregularity, cessation or retarded onset of periods, mood swings, depression, anxiety, reduction in breast or hip size, lack of, or fear of, sexual interest, and possible extra growth of body hair.

Predisposing factors

• Certain stresses and strains within the family group can contribute to problems in relation to food. Children of very competitive, appearance-conscious parents who may have problems of their own about weight, can have ambivalent feelings about food and eating habits.

• If an early sexual experience has been traumatic or distressing this can contribute to feelings of guilt and self-dislike, both of which can be common emotions experienced by those of us who have suffered from eating disorders.

• Shock or bereavement at a critical point of emotional or physical development, such as puberty.

Basic self-help measures

• Admit that a problem exists: once this is acknowledged, help and support can be given to overcome the situation.

• If the problem has become well established and long term, it will be helpful to seek the advice of a counsellor or psychotherapist who will be able to explore the psychological problems underlying the condition.

• Loneliness can support an environment where eating disorders will flourish: having the support and understanding of friends and a lively social life can help overcome an obsessive relationship with food.

- Gradually introduce small, extra helpings of nutritious food at each meal, or ensure that you have healthy snacks to hand, such as raw vegetables, rice cakes with cheese toppings, or ample portions of fresh fruit.

- Come to terms with reasons you may give for avoiding sitting down with family and friends for meals. Explore why this is necessary, and how you really feel about eating in the company of others.

- Keeping a diary can be an excellent way of recording your feelings so that you can obtain a long-term perspective on how your emotions affect the intensity of the problem you have in relation to food.

- Ensure that you are having adequate quantities of zinc in your daily intake of food. It has been suggested that there may be a link between low zinc levels in the body and eating disorders. Foods that contain this mineral include milk, eggs, green vegetables, wholegrains, yeast, meat, nuts and seeds.

Conventional treatment

Thankfully the days are now largely gone when anorexics were force-fed as in-patients in hospital. It has generally been acknowledged that this technique is extremely distressing and traumatic for the patient and is unlikely to help anyone come to terms with the psychological roots of their problem. In fact, it is far more likely that undergoing such an invasive procedure could lead to an increase in emotional distress, thus compounding the problem, rather than leading to a state of increased self-awareness. If someone has acknowledged that they are suffering from an eating disorder, they are now likely to be offered psychotherapy or psychiatric help.

Homoeopathic treatment

If an eating disorder is well established, homoeopathic treatment can have a vital role to play in helping the sufferer come to terms with their problem. Homoeopathic treatment can be very appropriately combined with counselling, emotionally supporting the client, encouraging and enabling them to come to terms with psychological insights as they arise. Self-medication is not appropriate for individuals suffering from eating disorders because of the complex psychological background to the condition. For this reason, the knowledge, objectivity and experience of a practitioner are needed in order to ensure that case management goes as smoothly as possible.

Insomnia

Sleep problems can vary from the very occasional bad night's sleep to regular and persistent insomnia. The variations within the insomniac state can also range from waking every hour or two after falling to sleep, to a severe problem with relaxing sufficiently in order to fall asleep initially. Problems can also include poor quality, light, unrefreshing sleep, or a tendency to feel wide awake and alert around dawn, but becoming exhausted later in the morning.

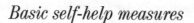

Basic self-help measures

- Make sure that the room is not too warm and stuffy or uncomfortably cold. Also check that the curtains block out light well.

- Avoid the trap of working very late at night. If your mind is still actively working on a problem it is very difficult to relax mentally and unwind sufficiently quickly for you to fall asleep. This is especially true before exams where the need for refreshing, good-quality sleep is increased.

- Make a habit of doing something relaxing for an hour or so before going to bed. This 'something' will vary from person to person: some of us might feel most relaxed after having a warm bath, while others might prefer to listen to music or read before falling asleep.

- Cut down, or cut out, strong tea, coffee and caffeinated fizzy drinks, especially during the evenings or at night. Symptoms that can arise from taking caffeine in regular quantities include: jitteriness and feeling on edge, rapid heartbeat, and general mental wakefulness and alertness at a time when the body wants to rest. Try alternative warm drinks at night, such as chamomile or fruit teas, coffee substitutes which are grain- or fig-based, or a warm milky drink (provided you do not suffer from catarrhal problems in the chest or sinuses, since dairy products can contribute to mucus production which is especially troublesome overnight).

- Avoid eating heavy, difficult-to-digest meals just before going bed.

- Experiment with essential oils that can help induce relaxation and sleep, such as lavender. You can add a few drops to the bath or your pillow, or even burn a small amount in a special holder in your bedroom. If you use essential oils, always remember that they are very concentrated and should not be used liberally: all you need are two or three drops at a time.

- Establish a pattern of regular exercise (ideally about three times a week) in order to give your mind and body a chance to deal with everyday stresses and strains. If this can include activity in the open air it will be extra beneficial in helping you to relax at night.

- Learn how to breathe in a way that encourages relaxation and helps diminish tension and anxiety. In order to do this, you need to learn how to breathe from your diaphragm (roughly from the area around your navel). Sitting in a high-backed chair, or lying down with your knees bent and feet on the floor, place your hand on your abdomen and relax, breathing out fully as you do so. As you breathe in, feel your hand lift gently as your abdomen expands after your chest has filled with air. Wait a second, then be aware of your abdomen flattening as you gently breathe out. Continue to breathe slowly, regularly and rhythmically in this way for as long as you feel comfortable. If you feel dizzy or light-headed, stop and breathe as you would normally until you feel clear-headed, and begin breathing from your diaphragm once more. You can use this invaluable tool to clear the mind and diminish panic whenever you are in a stressful situation, such as sitting an exam.

Conventional treatment

Your GP may prescribe a short course of sleeping pills if you are having sleeping problems due to anxiety about a specific event. However, the same drawbacks apply to long-term use of sleeping pills as to tranquillisers, and so it is more positive to consider alternative measures for coping such as hypnotherapy, herbalism or homoeopathy.

Homoeopathic treatment

If you are suffering from short-term insomnia within the context of normally sleeping soundly, it will be very helpful to use an appropriate homoeopathic remedy. This may sort out the short-term problem, enabling you to return to your normal, regular sleep pattern again. However, if you feel that insomnia is becoming a regular feature of your life, you need to seek professional help rather than attempting to deal with it yourself. A homoeopath will regard insomnia as a condition which needs constitutional treatment (treatment which is directed at improving your general state of health on all levels).

TYPE	GENERAL INDICATIONS	WORSE FROM	BETTER FOR	REMEDY NAME
Disturbed, light sleep after emotional stress or receiving distressing news	Spasmodic, violent yawning with inability to get to sleep. Bad dreams or recurrent nightmares. Jerking in limbs on falling asleep. Emotional strain and severe mood swings from lack of sleep.	Yawning. Bad news. Emotional strain	Being alone. Deep breathing. Changing position	Ignatia

TYPE	GENERAL INDICATIONS	WORSE FROM	BETTER FOR	REMEDY NAME
Sleep problems following a shock or trauma	Anxious, restless and panic-stricken with inability to sleep. Strong panic leads to conviction that death is near. Constantly tosses and turns in an effort to get settled. Disturbing dreams and nightmares on falling asleep. Often indicated after being involved in, or witnessing, an accident.	In bed. At night. Exposure to chill	Resting quietly. Fresh air	Aconite
Lack of sleep from physical over-tiredness	Difficulty in sleeping follows muscular strain, e.g. after a vigorous day's exercise overusing muscles that are not used to working. Bed feels too hard: tosses and turns all night in an effort to find a comfortable spot. Strong physical restlessness.	Touch. Muscular over-exertion	Lying with head lower than body	Arnica

TYPE	GENERAL INDICATIONS	WORSE FROM	BETTER FOR	REMEDY NAME
Lack of sleep from over-indulgence in food or alcohol	Very fitful, light sleep. Wakes between 3–4 a.m. Eventually falls asleep and does not want to get up when it is time to do so. Sleeplessness often follows abuse of caffeine when 'burning the candle at both ends' in an effort to cram in extra work. Irritable, oversensitive and argumentative with sleep problems.	Being disturbed. Stimulants. Exposure to cold or feeling chilled. Fuss	Being left in peace. Warmth in general. Warm drinks	Nux vomica
Difficulty getting to sleep before midnight	Mind refuses to switch off although very drowsy. Frustrated and irritable with sleeplessness. Very intolerant of overheated bedrooms. Recurrent thirst for cold drinks disturbs sleep. Mind preoccupied with work or domestic worries: dreams reflect these anxieties.	Early morning. Heat. Moving around. Being spoken to	Quiet. Cool. Cold drinks. Fresh air	Bryonia

TYPE	GENERAL INDICATIONS	WORSE FROM	BETTER FOR	REMEDY NAME
Anxious, disturbed sleep with tendency to wake between midnight and 2 a.m.	Terribly physically and mentally restless and agitated. May wake in a panic or with a start after falling asleep. Reacts very badly to cold environment and well to warmth in any form. Often feels more relaxed after a warm drink.	Chill and cold. Over tiredness. Midnight– 2 a.m. Being alone	Warmth. Warm drinks. Hot-water bottle. Company	Arsenicum album
Disturbed sleep from muscular aches and pains	Muscular pains brought on by over exertion or exposure to damp, cold. Tosses, turns and stretches constantly in an effort to get comfortable. Extreme physical restlessness with accompanying depression when wakeful.	After midnight. Keeping in one position. Resting. Exposure to damp, cold	Stretching. Limited movement. Warmth. Hot bathing	Rhus tox

If symptoms are persistent or if they do not respond to self-help measures, seek professional help.

Acne

Although acne is a condition that can strike at any stage of life, the teenage years are notorious for being the time when this distressing condition is most likely to surface. The misery that ensues can feel quite devastating when we are teenagers, since so much importance is put on our appearance at this time. Although skin conditions are often considered to be minor because they are not life-threatening, they can have a strongly negative effect on our quality of life, especially during stages in our lives when we feel self-conscious for a host of other reasons.

Although the severity of acne symptoms can vary from individual to individual, common symptoms of this condition include:

- Recurrent spots or pimples on chest, back, neck, chin, cheeks and forehead.

- Persistent oiliness affecting the areas mentioned above.

- Skin texture which is rather coarse with open pores and blackheads.

However, there are various positive steps that can be taken to help a great deal with this frustrating problem.

Basic self-help measures

- Avoid foods which have a reputation for aggravating skin conditions including acne. These include dairy products, such as full-fat milk and cheese, chocolate, fried foods and creamy cakes and sauces. Very sugary drinks and sweets may often result in a flare-up of the condition, while some sufferers find that they are very sensitive to citrus fruits, such as lemon, orange or grapefruit. If you suspect this may be the case, eliminate these fruits from your diet for a couple of months, and evaluate the quality of your skin over this period of time. If you have seen a definite improvement, re-introduce each citrus fruit slowly one at a time. If you experience a flare-up after introducing one of these fruits, eliminate it once again and give your skin a chance to settle down. Once things are stable again, re-introduce the fruit that you suspect caused a problem. If you observe an adverse reaction for the second time, you probably have a sensitivity to that food and should avoid it until your condition has improved greatly.

• Eat as many helpings of fresh fruit and vegetables as possible (ideally in their raw state). Remember to avoid citrus fruits if you suspect they may be aggravating your problem. Also make sure that you drink at least five to eight large glasses of spring or filtered water each day. This is one of the basic maintenance measures you can use to support your body's detoxifying capabilities. This is especially important if we bear in mind that our skin is one of the important routes that our bodies use to eliminate waste.

• Make sure that you have adequate supplies of vitamin C from your diet. Good sources include most raw fruit and vegetables. Bear in mind that vitamin C can be very easily destroyed by oxidation (leaving cut and peeled fruit or vegetables to sit for a while before eating), or by cooking, especially if vegetables are boiled for a long period of time. To preserve vitamin C content, eat fruit as soon as possible after it has been washed, peeled and cut, and eat vegetables raw, steamed or stir-fried in order to preserve their crispness.

• Avoid skin care products and make-up that may be aggravating your condition. Opt for formulas that are light and non-oily in texture, and do not make the mistake of cleansing your skin too frequently during the day. This can encourage oil production and make your skin even more sensitive. Also beware of harsh exfoliators which can irritate your skin further; it is wiser to choose clay- or mud-based exfoliators that can be gently removed by rolling movements over the skin. Choose cleansers that are specially formulated for oily or problem skins: these may be in the form of washes that can be lathered up with water and rinsed away, or light emulsions that can be removed with clean cotton wool. Follow with a toner to close the pores and finally apply a moisturiser that is specially formulated for oily, problem, or sensitive skins.

Conventional treatment

Possible options include antiseptic lotions and creams, or if symptoms are very severe, minor surgical techniques, such as dermabrasion, to remove scars. Long-term antibiotic therapy may be suggested, for instance taking Tetracycline tablets by mouth morning and evening.

Homoeopathic treatment

The following table contains a small selection of the potential range of homoeopathic medicines commonly used to treat sufferers from acne symptoms. There are tremendous advantages associated with holistic medical approaches in treating skin conditions, since they enable the patient to avoid the potential side-effects associated with conventional drugs such as antibiotics. Because homoeopaths regard skin conditions generally as a sign of a fundamental, systemic imbalance which needs to be addressed by

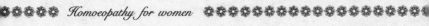

professional treatment, acne is a condition that should not be dealt with by home prescribing. However, if you suffer from the odd crop of spots from time to time, you will find the self-help measures outlined in the previous section, in combination with occasional doses of the appropriate homoeopathic remedy, may speed up the general healing process. However, if you start taking your homoeopathic remedy regularly in order to maintain an improvement, or if your symptoms are severe or very well established, it is necessary to seek professional advice.

TYPE	GENERAL INDICATIONS	WORSE FROM	BETTER FOR	REMEDY NAME
Spots on face that are much worse when anxious	Painful, inflamed spots that are soothed by warm applications and bathing, and worse for exposure to cold. Symptoms may emerge or be made very much worse for stress. Fussy and may become obsessed with keeping skin clean.	Cold. Alcohol. In winter	Warmth. Heat applied locally. Company	Arsenicum album
Eruptions on face which are very sensitive to touch	Very irritable and cold, sensitive with large spots rather like boils. Spots with pus formation and 'drawing' sensations. Tendency to dry, chapped skin which cracks easily. Cannot stand sensation of cold draughts on skin.	Touch. Pressure. Cold draughts. Dry, cold winds. In winter	Warmth. Humidity	Hepar sulph

TYPE	GENERAL INDICATIONS	WORSE FROM	BETTER FOR	REMEDY NAME
Initial stage of inflammation with localised heat and bright redness	Very intensely painful red spots which throb and radiate heat. Cannot stand touch, cold or jarring of sensitive areas. Inflammation develops rapidly with tremendous tenderness and general sense of irritability.	Touch. Lying on painful area. Jolting or jarring. Cold	Rest. Being left alone. Warmth	Belladonna
Acne which is worse before periods	Generally greasy skin on face with blackhead formation. Spots may be itchy and pronounced on cheeks and back. Skin is generally dry with a tendency to form cracks or cold sores, especially on the lips. Skin much worse for emotional stress and strain.	Before and after periods. Mental and emotional strain. Warmth. Touch. Sunlight	Cool bathing. Open air. Being left alone	Natrum mur
Blind spots on face with sweating and easy flushing	Pale, moist skin that goes red in warm surroundings, but also feels over sensitive to being cold. Easy weight gain from slow metabolic rate. Poor circulation, with constant sense of chilliness.	Being chilled. Contact with cold water. Before and during periods. Effort of any kind	Warmth. When constipated. Dry weather which is moderately warm	Calc carb

TYPE	GENERAL INDICATIONS	WORSE FROM	BETTER FOR	REMEDY NAME
Recurrent spots which heal very slowly and leave scars	Generally poor quality of skin, hair and nails which are brittle and break easily. Sweats easily around face and head. Tendency to boils which refuse to come to a head and resolve themselves. Skin is generally unhealthy and gets quickly infected.	Cold air. Pressure. Winter. Humidity	Warmth. Resting. Heat applied locally. Summer	Silica
Spots that emerge after eating too rich a diet, or emotional stress	Skin eruptions are much worse before periods and after eating chocolate or fatty foods. Feels much more comfortable when cool and much worse for heat in any form. Spots move from place to place or may affect one side of the body.	Being overheated. Stuffy rooms. Humidity. Resting. Feeling neglected	Fresh, open air. Gentle exercise. Cool applied locally. Having a good cry	Pulsatilla

If spots are becoming a long-term problem, or if you suspect there are signs of inflammation and infection of the skin, seek professional help.

Painful periods

Most young women suffer from painful periods in the first couple of years after their onset. This condition is often referred to as primary dysmenorrhoea. It is fortunate for

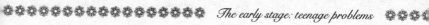

us that the severe pain often resolves itself by the time we reach our mid-twenties or after childbirth. The pain of menstruation can vary from person to person with some of us experiencing cramps and twinges that are easily coped with, and others going through a degree of pain that is so excruciating that it is impossible to function in a normal way. Apart from pain, the following symptoms can be attendant problems:

- Headaches and migraines.

- Extreme fatigue and weariness.

- Dizziness and fainting.

- Weepiness, irritability and abrupt mood swings.

- Vomiting and diarrhoea.

- Excessive perspiration.

Basic self-help measures

- If you suspect stress and emotional strain are factors which contribute to your problem, investigate ways of relaxing and unwinding.

- Make sure that your daily intake of food provides you with the necessary range of nutrients to maintain optimum health. Eat as many raw vegetables and fruit as possible, and avoid junk foods that are laden with fat and sugar. If you are considering using dietary supplements, appropriate possibilities include vitamins C, E, B-complex and Evening Primrose Oil.

- If you find heat soothing, relax in a warm bath as often as you can and apply warmth locally in the form of a heat pad or hot-water bottle.

• Increase the amount of exercise you take on a regular basis. Beneficial forms of exercise include vigorous aerobic activity to improve general circulation, such as running, swimming or cycling. Also experiment with stretching exercises that teach you how to relax specific muscle groups through breathing techniques.

• Use a TENS (transcutaneous electrical nerve stimulation) machine to provide effective and speedy pain relief. A TENS machine consists of two or four small pads attached to a battery operated unit. The pads are placed on the area where the pain is located and a very mild electrical current is passed between them. Once the user has adjusted the current to the point where they feel a mild tingling sensation, their pain subsides. The mechanism by which a TENS machine works is related to the 'gate' theory of pain relief. The latter is a concept whereby pain messages can be slowed down or stopped by low level stimulation involving mechanisms in the nervous system and the brain. When TENS is effective it has the tremendous advantage of providing rapid, effective pain relief without the side-effects associated with conventional painkillers.

Conventional treatment

Possibilities include the administration of drugs which inhibit the synthesis of prostaglandin (a substance which is believed to cause spasms of the muscles of the uterus). These drugs are usually taken from the onset of the pain for two or three days. A less popular approach to the problem is provided by prescribing the contraceptive pill as a means of suppressing ovulation.

Homoeopathic treatment

If painful periods have become a regular feature of every month, it is well worth seeking professional help from a homoeopath. Treatment will be aimed at bringing the body into a greater state of hormonal balance by prescribing on a 'constitutional' basis. It is also possible to provide acute, short-term pain relief by prescribing an appropriate homoeopathic remedy. Some of these are listed in the table below and may be useful in situations of acute pain. However, if symptoms are persistent, home-prescribing is not an appropriate substitute for professional treatment.

TYPE	GENERAL INDICATIONS	WORSE FROM	BETTER FOR	REMEDY NAME
Severe pain with profuse, bright red menstrual bleeding	Period may come too early with heavy, gushing, clotted flow that feels hot. Dragging pains with sensitive abdomen. Skin may be hot, dry and bright red with pain. Right-sided headache or migraine with period.	Motion. Jarring. Stimulation. Lying on painful part	Warmth. Resting. Keeping still	Belladonna

TYPE	GENERAL INDICATIONS	WORSE FROM	BETTER FOR	REMEDY NAME
Early onset of periods with labour-like pains	Flow is dark, profuse and contains large clots. Pains extend to the back and down the thighs. Hot, frantic and very bad-tempered with severe pain. Anger and frustration make pain worse. Strong cramping pains before and during period. Vomits with pain.	Heat. Draughts. Coffee. Before and during periods. Early part of the night	Moderate warmth	Chamomilla
Pain which is relieved as soon as flow is established	Strong pelvic pain for days before period comes: may be worse on the left side. Flow is heavy, dark and clotted. Dizzy before periods with left-sided headache. May feel flushed and sweaty with pain.	Tight clothes. Warm, stuffy rooms. Cold draughts. Waking from sleep. Touch. During puberty	Fresh, open air. Onset of menstrual flow and other discharges. Eating a little. Being active	Lachesis
Severe pains with vomiting and diarrhoea that are relieved by warmth	Chilly, pale, restless and anxious with pains. All symptoms feel much worse at night. Totally exhausted and prostrated with pains but cannot keep still because of mental and physical unease. Thirsty for small, frequent sips of warm drinks.	Cold in any form. Alcohol. At night. Any effort	Warmth. Warm drinks. Movement. Company	Arsenicum album

TYPE	GENERAL INDICATIONS	WORSE FROM	BETTER FOR	REMEDY NAME
Period pains with extreme sensitivity to cold and irritability	Nausea and vomiting with severe cramping pains which cause fainting. Bad-tempered and anxious before and during periods. Severe headaches or migraines. May be severely constipated with tenderness in abdomen. Pains are relieved by bending double.	Cold. Coffee or alcohol. Touch. Disturbed sleep. Mental effort. Mornings	Resting. Lying down. Unbroken sleep. As the day goes on. Firm pressure	Nux vomica
Late, scanty periods with weepiness	Nausea and vomiting accompany cutting pains that are worse for keeping still. Pains move about and constantly change in nature. Feels much worse for being alone and responds well to sympathy and attention. Although chilly, feels much worse for warm, airless rooms.	Night. Being alone. Warmth in any form. Lack of air. Keeping still. Being too warmly covered up	Gentle motion. Fresh, open air. Cool in any form. Sympathy and affection. Pressure	Pulsatilla

TYPE	GENERAL INDICATIONS	WORSE FROM	BETTER FOR	REMEDY NAME
Period pains with terrible nausea that is much worse from slightest movement	Awful nausea with pains that vomiting does not relieve. Very heavy flow that feels close to a haemorrhage. Bleeding is steady and bright red in colour or comes in gushes. Pains cause faintness and air hunger.	Extremes of heat or cold. Eating. Airless rooms. Movement of any kind	Fresh air. Keeping as still as possible. Firm pressure	Ipecac
Pains that are better from firm pressure or bending double	Waves of pain that come on abruptly and severely. Feels faint and weak but cannot keep still. Agitated, short-tempered and angry with pains: sends people away who try to help.	Cold. Anger. Iced drinks. Keeping still	Heat applied locally. Bending double. Firm pressure	Colocynthis
Delayed period with exhaustion and dragged-down sensations	Scanty flow with intense bearing-down sensations. Exhaustion worse in mornings. Feels as though everything is likely to fall out of pelvis: made worse by standing. Very depressed, apathetic and antisocial before and during period.	Before periods. Emotionally upset. Sitting still	Vigorous exercise. Open air. Being warm in bed. Eating. Sleep. Firm pressure	Sepia

If painful periods have become an established problem, or if pains are very severe, professional advice should be sought.

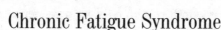

Chronic Fatigue Syndrome

This is a controversial condition that may be also referred to as ME (Myalgic Encephalomyelitis), Post Viral Syndrome, Royal Free Disease or Fibromyalgia. Conventional medical opinion is divided as to whether this condition exists or not, and varying theories have been put forward explaining the possible mechanisms that may be responsible for its development. However, there are a host of symptoms that sufferers of this syndrome may experience, including:

- Extreme fatigue and exhaustion on physical and mental levels.

- Muscle pains and weakness.

- Sleep disturbance.

- Headaches.

- Light and noise sensitivity.

- Glandular swelling and recurrent sore throats.

- Fluctuations in weight.

- Digestive problems such as loss of appetite and nausea.

- Mood swings including depression, weepiness, anxiety, irritability and panic when faced with stress.

Predisposing factors

- A viral illness such as a cold which has never fully cleared up and keeps relapsing.

- A stressful lifestyle which does not allow for time to

relax or unwind, combined with a tendency to 'burn the candle at both ends'. This often results in a dependence on stimulants to keep going during periods of extra stress e.g. during exams, and a generally poor quality diet lacking in essential nutrients.

• Chronic candida (thrush) infection.

• Repeated courses of drugs, such as antibiotics, that are thought to compromise the efficient functioning of our immune systems. It has also been suggested that some of us may also have an adverse reaction to vaccination, which can have long-term consequences with regard to the vigorous working of our immune systems.

Basic self-help measures

• Rest as much as possible in the early stages of being ill. Having ME means that the usual advice with regard to exercise stimulating energy levels does not apply. For an ME sufferer, increasing physical demands when exhausted will just make matters worse rather than better. As energy levels build up slowly, and provided the physical demands are well within the amount of energy available, it will be possible to become increasingly active. However, this must be taken slowly and steadily, and most important of all, the temptation to overdo things when energy levels are building should be resisted. Being patient in the early stages and working well within realistic limits can have a tremendously positive effect on stimulating an earlier recovery.

• Drink ten glasses of filtered or spring water each day

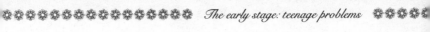

and ensure that you include as many whole foods in your daily intake as possible. Avoid convenience pre-packaged meals, refined sugar and flour in the form of biscuits and cakes, coffee, sugary fizzy drinks and alcohol.

• Consider supplementing with Evening Primrose Oil, and vitamins C, D and E. Some sources suggest that zinc deficiency may also be a co-factor for those who suffer ME. Where chronic candida infection is also present, garlic, acidophilus and Caprylic Acid supplements may also be helpful (See also section on self-help measures for **Thrush** in Chapter 3).

• As energy levels improve, begin to do some very gentle stretching exercises to help stimulate the lymphatic system. Take things very gently, beginning with some very simple yoga postures to loosen up your joints and help build muscle volume and strength.

• Experiment with visualisation exercises, meditation and relaxation techniques. Set aside some time each day in which to relax and concentrate on your breathing (see previous section on self-help measures for **Insomnia**).

• Use skin-brushing techniques to encourage detoxification. Using a natural bristle brush on dry skin (ideally before a bath or shower) brush firmly and gently in upward, sweeping movements, avoiding any areas where the skin may be irritated or broken.

Conventional treatment

There are conventional doctors who cannot accept that Chronic Fatigue Syndrome exists as an illness, but there are others who are firmly convinced that it does. The latter might suggest anti-depressants, ACE inhibitors (used to treat high blood pressure), anti-fungal preparations, such as Nystatin, or counselling. As yet, there is no accepted programme of treatment for Chronic Fatigue Syndrome or a definitive test to identify that the problem exists.

Homoeopathic treatment

Homoeopaths are regularly called upon to treat individuals with symptoms that suggest a diagnosis of ME. Because homoeopathy has at its core the notion that illness springs from a defence mechanism or immune system that has become overloaded with physical or emotional strain (or a potent combination of the two), we can see immediately that it is an appropriate therapeutic option for those who suffer from a problem such as ME. The bewildering range of symptoms that those ME patients experience also need not pose a particular problem to the homoeopath, since it is the latter's job constantly to identify the patterns that symptoms make in forming a whole symptom 'picture'. In other words, the homoeopath is constantly searching for the features in a group of symptoms that link them together in a coherent whole. Since homoeopathy, in common with other holistic approaches such as acupuncture, regards energy production as being a vital indicator of good, bad, or indifferent health, we can also see how it is especially well-placed to take on board the problems that ME sufferers experience. However, this is a condition where case management can be long, complicated, and fraught with relapses or set-backs. For these reasons, homoeopathic self-prescribing is not recommended in this situation.

Chronic Fatigue Syndrome is a condition which falls outside the scope of home prescribing and requires professional help.

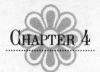

CHAPTER 4

THE INTERMEDIATE YEARS: MAKING THE MOST OF THEM

The information in this chapter covers some of the most common complaints that women experience during their twenties and thirties. Although not necessarily major in themselves, they can diminish our sense of pleasure and enjoyment in life. Many of these conditions can be dealt with through simple, self-help preventative measures which also improve our overall health. These basic suggestions for dietary, exercise and relaxation improvements are listed under the *Basic self-help measures* in each section.

By incorporating this advice into your daily routine, you will be surprised at the range of problems that seem to melt away into the background once the positive changes are established. You may also be delighted at the sense of satisfaction you experience when you have a range of self-help strategies at your disposal, rather than feeling unable to do anything positive when illness strikes.

For advice on how to use the remedy tables, please see the section entitled **Using this book: Selecting the right remedy** on page 19. To obtain the best results it is essential to read this information first and follow the directions as closely as possible, rather than attempting to use the tables without instructions.

Cystitis

Women are no strangers to the distressing problem of cystitis or bladder infections. It has been estimated that approximately three times more women than men suffer cystitis or urinary tract infections, and that forty per cent of women experience chronic (persistent or long-term) symptoms. Although varying in severity from individual to individual, and even from one attack to another, there are certain common symptoms we can use to identify cystitis or a urinary tract infection. These include:

- Frequency of urination.
- Discomfort ranging from a bearing-down sensation to excruciating burning pain on passing scanty amounts of urine.
- Abdominal bloating.
- Urine which is cloudy, dark, strong-smelling or bloody.
- If the infection travels from the bladder to the kidneys, symptoms may include pain in the lower back which radiates to the groin, feverishness, nausea or vomiting.

Predisposing factors

There are certain factors which can lead to an increased risk of developing or suffering recurrent bouts of cystitis. These include:

• Using a diaphragm that fits very snugly can inhibit the free flow of urine from the bladder. The presence of a diaphragm can also affect the bacterial balance in the vagina encouraging the growth of E. coli (one of the most common triggers of bladder infections).

• Recurrent thrush infection which also encourages the growth of E. coli.

• Wearing very tight clothing such as tight jeans, tights or leggings which create an environment favoured by bladder infections and thrush.

• Transferring bacteria from the anal region after passing a stool by wiping from back to front.

• Bladder infections often follow surgery which has called for catheterisation. This involves passing a small tube into the bladder to drain off urine when the patient cannot do so for herself, for example after a prolapse repair involving the bladder. As many as fifty per cent of infections acquired in hospital are urinary tract infections following catheterisation.

• Excess intake of irritants, such as caffeine or alcohol.

• Habitual constipation.

Basic self-help measures

All of the following measures will help to deal with an acute attack of cystitis and discourage its recurrence:

• Drink as much water as possible on a daily basis: at least eight large glasses a day. At the first sign of infection drink a large glass of water every hour until

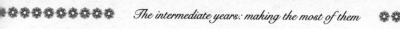

symptoms improve. Also drink cranberry juice every hour until discomfort has eased. Once symptoms are reduced, continue to drink cranberry juice twice a day until you are confident that the infection has gone completely.

• You can make your own barley water by boiling pearl barley in a pan of water and straining off the liquid which can be cooled and stored in the fridge. Unlike commercially prepared barley waters, which include citrus juice (orange or lemon) and a high proportion of sugar (both of which further irritate the bladder), home-made barley water reduces the acidity of the urine, making it less painful to pass.

• During an acute attack try to rest as much as possible and experiment with warm or cool applications to the lower abdomen to see which is more soothing.

• Avoid alcohol, citrus fruits, sweetened carbonated drinks and caffeine while symptoms are present. If you suffer from chronic cystitis (frequent or long-term bouts of infection) it is good to avoid the former as much as possible.

• Cut down on the amount of sugar in your diet and concentrate on fresh fruit (avoiding grapes, citrus fruit and strawberries), and fresh vegetables (avoiding tomatoes, spinach, asparagus, potatoes and raw carrots). Other foods to concentrate on include whole grains, unsaturated fats and protein that is low in fat, including poultry and fish.

• Ensure you do not suffer from constipation by including enough water and fibre in your diet.

• Wear natural fibres such as cotton rather than nylon around the groin area and avoid wearing tights or very tight trousers every day.

• Drink water and empty your bladder before intercourse. If you are subject to repeated bouts of cystitis, washing gently with warm water after intercourse (avoiding perfumed soap or bubble bath) will help discourage re-infection.

• Never ignore the impulse to pass water: try to pass water every few hours and ensure that you completely empty your bladder each time.

• After passing a stool always wipe from front to back rather than vice versa.

• Consider supplementing with garlic. This has a reputation for combating a broad spectrum of micro-organisms, including those which may lead to urinary tract infections. Choose a brand which provides concentrated, odourless garlic: this is a definite bonus if you or your family and friends cannot stand its smell!

• You may also benefit from a course of vitamin C as a general preventative measure against infection. However, high doses (a gram or more a day) should be avoided over sustained periods of time since this may encourage kidney stone formation.

Conventional treatment

This will usually consist of a prescription for antibiotics. If the problem has become long term with attacks recurring at frequent or regular intervals, some investigative procedures may be suggested, such as an X-ray of the bladder or the kidneys, in order to check for functional problems.

Homoeopathic treatment

The following are suggestions of appropriate homoeopathic remedies which can be used to treat the isolated or very infrequent attack of cystitis. When used effectively the appropriate homoeopathic remedy can provide swift relief of symptoms without the risk of setting off a bout of thrush. Unfortunately, many women have found the latter can occur after a course of antibiotics. If you suffer from long-term attacks it is wise to seek professional advice.

TYPE	GENERAL INDICATIONS	WORSE FROM	BETTER FOR	REMEDY NAME
Cystitis with stinging pains which are much worse from warmth	Terrible burning, stinging pains that are much better for cool applications. Very restless and irritable with pains. Thirstless with cystitis. Urine feels scalding and must be passed immediately. Fluid retention with symptoms.	Warmth. Pressure. Touch. Lying down. At night	Cool in any form. Movement. Open air	Apis mellifica

TYPE	GENERAL INDICATIONS	WORSE FROM	BETTER FOR	REMEDY NAME
Cystitis with severe burning pains that are much relieved by warmth	Generally chilly, restless, anxious and unwell with cystitis. May be nauseated. Feels much better for sipping warm drinks, applying a hot-water bottle or warm compresses to sensitive areas, and staying in a warm room.	Cold rooms. During the night. Alcohol	Warmth. Sips of warm drinks. Company. Sweating	Arsenicum album
Sudden onset of cystitis with violent, burning pains	Exhausted with cystitis. Pains are felt before, during and after passing very small amounts of scalding urine. Constant desire to pass water. Pains may extend to the kidneys. Generalised sensation of burning with shivering and chilliness.	Movement. Touch. Drinking. Coffee	Warmth. At night	Cantharis
Stinging pains with concentrated, dark-coloured urine that is difficult to pass	Symptoms may follow sexual activity or catheterisation. Burning during passage of urine which continues even after bladder has been emptied. Distressed by a constant sensation of incomplete urination. Very irritable and bad-tempered with symptoms.	Slight touch. Pressure. Intercourse. Early morning	Warmth. Resting. After eating	Staphysagria

66

TYPE	GENERAL INDICATIONS	WORSE FROM	BETTER FOR	REMEDY NAME
Fever with cystitis: symptoms develop with extreme rapidity and violence	Generally hot and irritable: skin feels dry and burning to the touch. Very sensitive to movement: especially jarring. Symptoms may be aggravated by pregnancy. Blood may be present in urine. Although drowsy and wanting to sleep, insomnia is persistent.	Stimulation. Noise. Bright light. Jolting	Warm rooms. Resting. Keeping still. Sitting propped-up in bed	Belladonna
Cystitis that is brought on by getting cold and wet, or becoming chilled after being overheated	Frequent need to pass water that must be acted on immediately: if not, urine is passed involuntarily. Thrush may accompany cystitis. Discomfort continues after passing water. Cannot lie on the back without needing to pass water. Weepy and in need of a lot of sympathy and attention.	Stuffy rooms. At night. Warmth. Resting	Open; fresh air. Cool in general. Gentle exercise. Sympathy	Pulsatilla

TYPE	GENERAL INDICATIONS	WORSE FROM	BETTER FOR	REMEDY NAME
Cystitis with marked irritability and sensitivity to cold	Constant desire to pass water with terrible difficulty in doing so. Burning sensations in bladder at night with itching or burning on passing water. Even if very hot, cannot put a hand or foot outside bedcovers without feeling uncomfortable. Cystitis may follow 'burning the candle at both ends' and relying on stimulants to keep the pace.	Cold draughts. Stimulants. Coffee. Spicy foods. Touch. Disturbed sleep. On waking	Undis-turbed napping. Resting. As the day goes on	Nux vomica
Anxiety and digestive problems with cystitis	Lots of bloating, wind and general abdominal discomfort: needs to loosen waistband in order to be comfortable. Very stressed and anxious with cystitis. Aching in back and sides before passing water which feels better afterwards. Flow of urine may take a long time to get started.	Stress. Hot, stuffy rooms. Getting too cold. On waking and in the afternoon	Being comfortably warm. Warm drinks. Being occupied. Open air	Lycopodium

TYPE	GENERAL INDICATIONS	WORSE FROM	BETTER FOR	REMEDY NAME
Cystitis with incontinence of urine when coughing or sneezing	Symptoms develop slowly and insidiously with general feeling of being 'run down'. Pains feel sore, raw or tearing, leaving area affected very sensitive to any contact. Urine may be passed involuntarily at night.	Exposure to dry, cold winds. After bathing. Movement. Coffee. Getting wet	Warmth. In bed	Causticum

Seek professional advice if:

- you have pain in your kidneys;

- there is blood in your urine;

- you are vomiting or have a high temperature

- symptoms persist and do not respond to self-help measures.

Thrush

Women are frequent sufferers of vaginal thrush and many have suffered the problem as a result of taking antibiotics for a bout of cystitis. As a result, a vicious circle can be set up where the drug treatment for urinary tract infections can lead to recurrent problems with thrush requiring separate medication. The reason for the problem is now well known: antibiotics promote the overgrowth of *candida albicans*, a yeast-like fungus that lives happily in the digestive tract provided it is kept in check by other bacteria. However, if the balance of the intestinal flora is disturbed though antibiotic therapy, candida can spread outside the gut wall. This overgrowth can lead to the symptoms the majority of us are familiar with as thrush. These symptoms include:

- Vaginal itching, dryness and soreness which are often aggravated during sexual intercourse. The discomfort can be so severe in some cases that it makes intercourse impossible or extremely undesirable.

- A thick, white, cottage cheese like discharge that may smell yeasty.

- A red scaly rash may extend to the upper, inner sides of the thighs.

- Frequent urination with stinging on passing water.

General symptoms of candida overgrowth can also include the following:

- Digestive problems, such as constipation, diarrhoea, abdominal bloating or low blood sugar levels.

- Cystitis.

- Pre-menstrual Syndrome (PMS) including water retention, mood swings, breast tenderness and enlargement, and exhaustion.

- Food sensitivities.

- Joint problems.

- Chronic fatigue.

- Skin rashes.

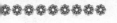
Predisposing factors

These include:

- Recent treatment with antibiotics.

- Use of the contraceptive pill.

- A diet which is high in refined carbohydrates (white sugar and flour).

- Women who have high progesterone levels, for example, before a period or during pregnancy.

- A history of diabetes.

Basic self-help measures

- Avoid sugar, alcohol and refined carbohydrates, such as white bread, vinegar and junk foods. Concentrate on whole foods, fish, fresh vegetables, fruit, and as much filtered water as possible.

- Consider supplementing with garlic tablets. Take two tablets three times a day.

- If symptoms are chronic, consider using an acidophilus, caprylic acid, or essential fatty acid (evening primrose oil or linseed oil) supplement. Also include live natural yoghurt in your diet.

- For an acute attack douche with a solution of vinegar and water or take a salt bath. Live natural yoghurt can also be immensely soothing if applied to the vagina.

- Avoid highly scented bubble baths, vaginal deodorants, tight-fitting nylon underwear, tights and tampons.

Wear loose cotton underwear and avoid tight jeans during an acute bout of thrush. Check that you do not have a sensitivity to condoms, your diaphragm or contraceptive gel or cream.

• Do not use creams which contain a local anaesthetic: these will merely mask the symptoms for a very short time and you may develop a sensitivity to them.

Conventional treatment

A swab may be taken to confirm that you are suffering from a candida infection. If confirmed, treatment usually consists of anti-fungal pessaries and/or cream. If the infection refuses to clear or re-occurs, you may be offered anti-fungal tablets to take by mouth.

Homoeopathic treatment

The remedies suggested below are the most commonly indicated homoeopathic medicines for treating an isolated bout of thrush. If you select the one which matches your own symptoms most closely you will find it soothes and eases itching and discomfort decisively and rapidly. However, if you suspect you are suffering from a systemic candida infection, or are experiencing repeated bouts of thrush, it is wise to seek professional help to ensure the most positive outcome. It is also best to avoid using Calc Carb or Sulphur too frequently: these are both very deep-acting remedies that have a slow-developing action. For this reason wait longer between doses in order to assess whether a curative response has been activated. If in doubt, always pause rather than routinely re-prescribing.

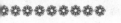

TYPE	GENERAL INDICATIONS	WORSE FROM	BETTER FOR	REMEDY NAME
Thrush with burning sensation that is eased by warmth	Restlessness, anxiety and chilliness with feeling unwell. Itching and burning are eased by warmth and warm applications. Thin, watery discharge which is stinging, burning and smarting.	At night. Cold in any form. Alcohol	Warmth. Heat applied locally. Warm drinks. Moving about	Arsenicum album
Thrush with creamy, bland, or yellowish-green discharge	Symptoms are worse before a period or during pregnancy. Weepiness and a need for sympathy accompany feeling unwell. Feels better for keeping cool and much worse for warmth. Thrush may be brought on by puberty.	Warmth. Stuffy rooms. In the evening. Keeping still. Becoming heated in bed	Sympathy. Attention. Gentle exercise. Cool, fresh air. Uncovering	Pulsatilla
Thrush with irritating, thick, offensive yellowish-green discharge	Depression, irritability and exhaustion accompany feeling ill. Everything feels worse in the morning. Constipation occurs with thrush. Dry sensation of vagina with aversion to intercourse.	Before a period. Emotional demands. Sitting still	Vigorous exercise. Taking a nap. Open, fresh air. Warmth. Afternoons	Sepia

TYPE	GENERAL INDICATIONS	WORSE FROM	BETTER FOR	REMEDY NAME
Thrush with sour-smelling, thick, profuse discharge	Completely exhausted and washed-out with symptoms that keep recurring. Itching, burning and smarting accompany a thick discharge that may be worse before and during a period. Craves sweet foods or dairy products.	Getting chilled. Cold draughts. Bathing. At night. Over-exertion	Warmth. Being constipated	Calc carb
Thrush which occurs at ovulation (mid-way through menstrual cycle)	Bland or irritating discharge that feels like warm water and looks clear or like egg white. Thrush occurs before or after period. Swelling, itching and burning in vagina.	Warmth. After periods. Touch		Borax
Thrush with very offensive greenish discharge that is much worse at night	Very restless, distressed and uncomfortable for being warm in bed at night. Severe insomnia from discomfort with strong sensitivity to cold draughts. Severe itching is relieved by cold bathing and discharge may be increased when passing water.	At night. Extremes of heat or cold. Becoming warm in bed. At night. In the evening. Touch. Sweating	Resting. Moderate temperatures	Mercurius

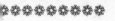

TYPE	GENERAL INDICATIONS	WORSE FROM	BETTER FOR	REMEDY NAME
Thrush with fluent discharge that looks like uncooked egg-white	Very depressed, weepy and low-spirited with a strong aversion to sympathy and fuss. Symptoms may follow on from stress, shock or suppressed feelings. May have recurrent tendency to cold sores when health is under strain. Vaginal pain during intercourse.	During or after a period. Warmth. Stuffy rooms. Touch. Sympathy and attention. After sleep	Open, fresh air. Not eating. Cool bathing. Gentle exercise	Natrum mur
Thrush which is aggravated by becoming chilled, and before periods	Frequent urge to pass water and general soreness in vagina. Swollen, painful breasts before period. Symptoms may follow a stressful, anxious or depressing time. Weary, shivery and chilly when ill. General tendency to low back pain.	Cold air. Least touch. Coffee. Exertion. Becoming overheated	During the day. Warmth. Open air	Kali carb

TYPE	GENERAL INDICATIONS	WORSE FROM	BETTER FOR	REMEDY NAME
Thrush with terrible itching, burning pain and heavy discharge that are worse during the week before period is due	Discharge may be yellow or white and very offensive. Marked itching which is made much worse for exposure to heat in any form. Persistent headaches accompany symptoms: these may be much worse before a period. Symptoms may be aggravated during the menopause. Itching may extend to anus from vagina.	Heat. In bed at night. Mid-morning. Bathing. Severe cold	Moderate temperature	Sulphur

Seek professional advice if:

• Symptoms refuse to respond to self-help measures within a few days or if you experience recurrent bouts of the problem.

Pre-Menstrual Syndrome (PMS)

The symptoms of PMS can vary in nature and degree. Many women find they suffer from a range of symptoms during the second half of their menstrual cycle. These can include:

• Pains at ovulation (mid-cycle).

• Tender and enlarged breasts.

- Fluid retention: especially around the waist and abdomen.

- Cravings for sweet foods and stimulants.

- Sleep disturbance.

- Strong and unpredictable mood swings including weepiness, irritability, depression, lack of confidence and feelings of self-destruction.

- Severe period pains.

- Lack of co-ordination.

- Pre-menstrual headaches.

- Thrush and/or cystitis.

- Skin disorders, such as acne.

As we can see from the list given above, the range of potential symptoms suffered by those of us who suffer PMS is immense. When we add into the equation that some of us feel our symptoms are so intense and severe that we only experience two balanced and creative weeks out of every four, it is apparent that this is a serious problem that demands effective action.

Predisposing factors

- A diet which is high in convenience foods. These generally include a high proportion of sodium (which makes fluid-retention worse), refined carbohydrates, sugar, and an array of chemical colourings and additives. Including regular amounts of alcohol in the diet can also lead to vitamin deficiencies, especially if you smoke, drink strong tea and coffee and take the contraceptive pill.

• A high daily intake of dairy foods.

• A history of hormone imbalance or chronic candida problems.

• A tendency to low blood sugar levels (hypoglycaemia).

Basic self-help measures

• Include as many whole, unrefined foods as possible in your diet, including whole grains, a high proportion of fresh, raw vegetables and fruit in the form of salads, at least six large glasses of filtered water daily, and ensure that you have adequate amounts of protein from low fat sources, such as fish or poultry (using white meat). If you are a vegetarian make sure that you are having enough complete protein by combining pulses and cereals together during a meal.

• Consider supplementing with vitamin C, B-complex (rather than taking isolated components of this complex in isolation), Evening Primrose Oil, or a good quality multi vitamin and mineral combination. This is very important if you suspect your diet does not include enough fresh, raw foods.

• Avoid salted foods by adding other flavourings to your foods to ensure that they do not taste bland. Possibilities include toasted herbs or ground, toasted sunflower seeds.

• Cut down on the amount of sugar in your diet by

eliminating extra sources such as fizzy drinks. Instead use unsweetened fruit juices, such as apple, or one of the more exotic combinations that are now available. Substitute fresh fruit for puddings where possible, or eat live yoghurt. Use dried fruit, sunflower seeds or unsalted nuts occasionally as a snack (try to obtain fruit that has not been treated with sulphur dioxide).

• Cut down on tea and coffee by using some of the very palatable herbal combinations that are now available. Drink these warm, or, if you prefer, make up a pint of the drink and put it in the fridge to cool. You can then serve it chilled in a long glass.

• Find a form of exercise that you enjoy and include it in your weekly schedule. The ideal to work towards is one half hour session at least three times a week, but not more than five. However, don't be put off even if you can only initially manage half an hour a week: this is better than nothing. Regular, rhythmical exercise helps discourage fluid retention, boosts energy levels and can help diminish feelings of depression.

• Explore relaxation techniques, meditation, or diaphragmatic breathing. All of these can help deal with feeling stressed, irritable or anxious, especially when combined with regular exercise.

• If you suspect you suffer from low blood sugar levels (symptoms include light-headedness, dizzy spells, nausea and general fatigue) make sure that you eat small amounts every two hours. You may need no more than a piece of fruit or a slice of bread to keep your blood sugar levels steady, but eat it all the same. Avoid foods that encourage peaks and troughs of blood sugar levels:

these include strong tea and coffee, and sugary foods such as cakes, biscuits, chocolate or very sweet carbonated drinks.

Conventional treatment

Depending on the severity and range of the symptoms and the approach of your GP, treatment could include diuretics (these stimulate urine production in an effort to control water retention), progesterone, doses of vitamin B6, Evening Primrose Oil, painkillers, antidepressants, tranquillisers, counselling or psychotherapy.

Homoeopathic treatment

If you suffer from minor symptoms on an irregular basis, one of the following homoeopathic medicines could be of tremendous help in allieviating your problem, especially if you also employ the self-help measures suggested above. Remember that homoeopathic medicines are not designed to be taken on a long-term basis: two or three doses taken over one or two days should be all you need.

However, if you are suffering from a wide range of severe symptoms every month, it is best to seek professional help and advice. Homoeopathy and other holistic methods of healing have a tremendous amount to offer in treating PMS since they emphasise the need to treat the whole person. As a result, emotional disturbances are evaluated within the overall context of energy levels and general well-being. Treatment is aimed at elevating the experience of health on all levels, mental, emotional, and physical, rather than being solely concerned with the removal of isolated symptoms. When successful, the end result is a qualitative difference in experience of health.

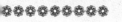

TYPE	GENERAL INDICATIONS	WORSE FROM	BETTER FOR	REMEDY NAME
Symptoms of PMS that are improved as soon as flow begins	Violent mood swings and terrible insomnia in days leading up to period. All symptoms are much worse waking from sleep. Left-sided headaches, migraines and ovarian pain. Cramping pains that are relieved as soon as the period begins. Clotting or flooding with dark menstrual bleeding.	Becoming overheated. Hot bathing. Cold draughts. Touch. Tight clothing. Before a period	Open, fresh air. Onset of discharges. Eating moderate amounts. Movement. Once menstrual flow begins	Lachesis
PMS with breasts enlarged, tender breasts and extreme tiredness	Exhaustion during days leading up to period, with chilliness, fluid retention, constipation and weight gain. Cravings for sweets, dairy foods and indigestible things. Totally exhausted with a tendency to clammy sweat when making an effort. Anxious, fearful and panicky before periods.	Cold and damp. Cold bathing. Being overtired. Fresh air	Warmth. Being constipated. Lying down	Calc carb

TYPE	GENERAL INDICATIONS	WORSE FROM	BETTER FOR	REMEDY NAME
Exhaustion, irritability and profound depression with PMS	Feels everything is drooping downwards. Moods alternate between screaming, violence, weeping and emotional withdrawal. General weariness with lack of interest in sex. Bearing-down pains in lower abdomen with possible prolapse of the uterus. PMS worse after childbirth.	Before, during or after period. Not eating. Touch. Mornings. Resting	Eating. Vigorous exercise, such as aerobics or dancing. Running or fast walking. Raising legs	Sepia
PMS with strong need for attention and sympathy	Oversensitive, weepy and sad state which is relieved by having a good cry. Although chilly, feels much worse for being in warm, stuffy rooms and better for open air. Craves company and attention, which has a very positive effect. Chronic tendency to vaginal infections and irritation, such as thrush. Indigestion, nausea, vomiting, headaches, diarrhoea and back pain may happen before or during periods.	Stuffy, airless rooms. Being overheated. Resting. At night. Rich or fatty foods. Feeling neglected	Gentle exercise. Fresh, open air. Cool applications. Pressure. Sympathy. Weeping	Pulsatilla

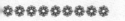

TYPE	GENERAL INDICATIONS	WORSE FROM	BETTER FOR	REMEDY NAME
Depression and inward sadness which are made worse by sympathy and attention	Withdrawn mental state and repressing of emotion with intolerance of consolation. Crying provides no release and makes everything feel worse. Fluid retention, severe headaches or migraines and skin rashes or cold sores are common before or after periods. Dry skin and cracked lips occur when feeling run down. Craving for salty foods.	Consolation. Attention. Crying. Direct sunlight or becoming overheated. Noise. Touch or pressure	Going without meals. Cool bathing. Resting. Open, fresh air	Natrum mur
PMS with reliance on alcohol and stimulants to keep going	Irritability, headaches, indigestion and constipation before periods. Strong craving for caffeine, strong-flavoured foods, cigarettes and alcohol in order to cope with stress. Symptoms of workaholism get worse before periods with marked tendency to insomnia. Dizziness, backache, joint pains and general muscular tension.	Stress. Interrupted sleep. Cold draughts. Being chilled. Stimulants. Touch	Warmth. Rest. Unbroken sleep. As the day goes on. Firm pressure	Nux vomica

TYPE	GENERAL INDICATIONS	WORSE FROM	BETTER FOR	REMEDY NAME
Marked irritability and depression before period with disturbed digestion	Insecurity and anxiety pre-menstrually, especially if asked to speak in public. Depression lifts once flow begins. Painful heavy periods with dark, clotted flow. Feels as though gas is being passed through vagina. Very bloated, rumbling abdomen with constipation. Indigestion and bilious attacks with craving for sweet things. Always feels worse in afternoons.	Cold air. Exertion. Cold drinks. Being overheated. Tight clothes around waist. Windy foods such as pulses, beans and cabbage	Warmth. Fresh air. Gentle motion out of doors. Loosening clothing	Lycopodium
Exhaustion, chilliness and marked fluid retention before periods	Insomnia, panic attacks and general state of tension before periods. Breast enlargement and tenderness and constipation with backache. Marked swelling of waterlogged tissues, especially around upper eyelids. General tendency to catarrhal conditions and sinusitis.	Early morning. Cold draughts. Coffee. Least touch or pressure	Warmth. During the day. Open air. Sitting bending forwards	Kali carb

Seek professional advice if:

- Symptoms are severe and well established.

- Self-help measures have not been of help.

- Emotional symptoms are severe.

- Bleeding or 'spotting' occurs between periods.

- Sexual intercourse becomes painful.

Endometriosis

Endometriosis is a distressing chronic condition that has a reputation for affecting women from their late twenties through their reproductive years. The problem occurs when small cysts of endometrial tissue (the endometrium being the lining of the womb) migrate to other areas including the ovaries, inside the muscle of the womb, or the pelvis. They bleed at the time of menstruation, but because there is no outlet for the bleeding, the cysts stretch and become painful. It can take a long time before symptoms arise: often up to ten or fifteen years. Once problems arise, they can include:

- Lower abdominal pain.

- Very painful periods.

- Infertility.

- Pain during intercourse.

- Depression

- Fluid retention and weight gain.

- Breast tenderness.

- Nausea, burning on passing urine, irritability or weepiness before periods.

- Endometriosis can sometimes be symptomless.

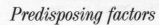

Predisposing factors

Endometriosis has traditionally been regarded as a disease associated with career women, especially if they choose not to have children. While the career factor is now seen as being less relevant, the option of remaining childless (or being infertile) still seems to be relevant. Age also plays its part, since young women in their early twenties are less likely to suffer with endometriosis, while women in their thirties and forties are most likely to exhibit symptoms. Contributing factors may include selenium deficiency and the use of tampons.

Basic self-help measures

See the measures suggested in the PMS section. Although endometriosis is a chronic condition that requires professional help, many of these adjunctive suggestions may be useful.

Conventional treatment

Endometriosis is diagnosed after a laparoscopy (a surgical procedure where a small telescope is inserted into the abdomen through a tiny incision in the navel under anaesthetic) to identify if the small cysts are present. If the findings are positive, treatment may consist of an oral contraceptive, or danazol, which inhibits ovulation. If the condition is not extensive it may be practical to have the cysts removed surgically. However, if the problem has become widespread and the cysts are too numerous to be removed, a hysterectomy may be suggested.

Homoeopathic treatment

Because endometriosis is a deep-seated, chronic condition, it is essential that professional help is sought. In conditions such as these, self-help is unlikely to yield anything more than very short-term relief at best. A homoeopath, on the other hand, will be able to prescribe on a 'constitutional' basis, taking into account all the predisposing factors in the development of the problem.

Anyone who is suffering from endometriosis should seek professional advice.

Migraines

It has been estimated that as many as seventy per cent of migraine sufferers are women. Fortunately, many of us will outgrow the tendency once we have experienced the menopause. This is very good news, since anyone who has suffered a severe migraine will be aware of how disabling a condition this can be, especially if attacks occur at regular intervals interrupting time spent relaxing with families or work patterns.

It is important to identify the difference between a classic migraine and a headache, since there can be as much confusion around classifying these two conditions as there is between distinguishing an episode of flu from the common cold. The common symptoms of migraine include:

- Visual disturbance or an 'aura' (zig-zag patterns or flashing lights before the eyes) which often is the first sign of an approaching migraine.

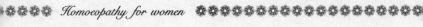

- A sense of confusion, disorientation, slurred speech or lack of co-ordination.

- Pain which often begins at the back of the head and may radiate above, or behind the eyes. This often affects one side of the head.

- Nausea, vomiting, and diarrhoea.

- Tingling and numbness of the limbs.

- Intolerance to light.

Migraine sufferers can experience any combination of these symptoms in varying severity, and in any order. However, the common pattern is often visual disturbance, followed by pain, nausea and vomiting. This will generally subside after a day or so, leaving the sufferer feeling washed out and generally fragile for anything between twenty-four to forty-eight hours.

Predisposing factors

- Taking the contraceptive pill may aggravate symptoms.

- A poorly-aligned jaw or grinding teeth at night may contribute to the problem.

- Eye or sinus problems.

- A stressful lifestyle with little time for relaxation.

- Low blood sugar levels.

- High blood pressure.

- Working for long periods of time at a VDU screen without sufficient breaks.

- Many migraine sufferers have inherited a familial tendency to develop the condition.

Basic self-help measures

- Make relaxation techniques or meditation an integral part of your day. This may involve no more than ten or twenty minutes of your time, but the benefits are enormous. It is more important to aim for regularity than length of time spent relaxing each day. Most important of all, this will give you a sense that this is a part of your time that is devoted to yourself, away from the demands of work or family. To achieve this, you ideally need the co-operation of your partner and family, so that it is understood that this is a time of day when you are not to be disturbed. Otherwise, ensure that you unplug your telephone and sit or lie down in the most quiet room you have.

- Exercise is also an essential way of reducing stress, clearing the mind and increasing our energy levels and vitality. Choose whatever activity you find most fun and enjoyable: it is essential you choose something which is not boring or it will be very hard to maintain your enthusiasm. Consider yoga as an activity that encourages our bodies to develop and improve suppleness and stamina, while also teaching us how to breathe in a way that enhances relaxation.

- Having a regular massage is an excellent way of encouraging tense muscles to relax and encouraging a general sense of tranquillity and well-being.

- Certain foods seem to make migraines worse. These include: coffee, chocolate, cheese, alcohol (especially red wine and gin), tea, citrus fruits, wheat, cured meats, such as salami and bacon, pork and shellfish. If you suspect one of these might be a factor, eliminate it from your diet for a month and evaluate any changes during that time. If when you re-introduce the item you experience a problem, it is well worth avoiding that food.

• Consider taking a vitamin C and B-complex supplement, especially if you take the contraceptive pill or if you smoke. Evening Primrose Oil may also be helpful.

• Avoid low blood sugar levels by eating small amounts regularly and eliminating foods and drinks that play havoc with blood sugar. These include coffee, refined sugary foods, such as biscuits and cakes, and chocolate. Substitute small pieces of fruit or raw vegetables instead.

• Avoid getting constipated by incorporating enough fibre in your diet through whole grains, fresh, raw vegetables and fruit.

Conventional treatment

The medication that may be used to treat migraines can include any of the following: antihistamines, vasoconstrictors, anti-emetics, antidepressants, tranquillisers, or anti-hypertensives. Those doctors who are interested in a more holistic approach may suggest cranial osteopathy, dental attention to deal with misalignment of the jaw, or biofeedback to aid relaxation.

Homoeopathic treatment

The medicines listed below can give effective, short-term pain relief during an attack of migraine, provided you identify the most appropriate medicine for your individual symptoms. However, they are unlikely to be able to deal with your susceptibility to the problem because migraines are a chronic problem. For the most positive outcome it is wise to seek help from a trained homoeopath who will be able to see your migraines within the broader context of your overall health. Homoeopathic treatment has an enormous amount to offer in the treatment of migraine by easing pain, shortening attacks and enabling the sufferer to recover more quickly. It has the added bonus of offering treatment which does not have the side-effects of the conventional medication used to treat this condition.

On the other hand, if you suffer from occasional headaches, you will find the information included in the table below invaluable in enabling you to identify the most appropriate remedy to ease the pain and resolve the problem.

TYPE	GENERAL INDICATIONS	WORSE FROM	BETTER FOR	REMEDY NAME
Left-sided migraines which are much worse on waking	Base of the skull is tender to touch and scalp may also be very tender. Throbbing pains above the left eye extend to the bridge of the nose. Migraine may come on after exposure to cold or direct sunlight.	After sleep. In the morning. Before a period. Touch	Lying down. Warmth. Nasal discharge. Open air	Lachesis

TYPE	GENERAL INDICATIONS	WORSE FROM	BETTER FOR	REMEDY NAME
Migraines that are prompted by sensitivity to alcohol	Heavy sensation in head with nausea and constipation. May feel that vomiting would help, but cannot. Very irritable and oversensitive on emotional and physical levels. Cannot tolerate interruption, noise or being disturbed. Also terribly sensitive to draughts of cold air.	Excitement. Cold in general. Draughts of cold air. Noise. On waking, especially first thing in the morning. Coffee and other stimulants	Warmth. Rest. Undisturbed sleep. As the day goes on	Nux vomica
Migraines that are preceded by numbness or tingling in the face	Visual disturbance may be the first indicator of a developing migraine. Accompanied by, or closely followed by numbness and tingling of the face, lips and cheeks. Very dry tongue and terrific thirst before an attack. Sensations in head may be throbbing or burning and relieved by lying down. Attack may be set off by stress, grief, unexpressed emotion or travel sickness.	Moving eyes. Sunlight. Before, or during a period. Hot, stuffy rooms. Touch or pressure. After sleep (may sometimes help)	Open air. Lying down. Missing meals. Cool bathing	Natrum mur

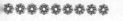

TYPE	GENERAL INDICATIONS	WORSE FROM	BETTER FOR	REMEDY NAME
Migraine with exhaustion and droopy, heavy sensation in limbs	Dimness of vision precedes an attack. Pain spreads from back of neck to forehead with a sensation of a vice or tight band above the eyes. Right-sided pain. Droopy eyelids: looks washed-out. Just wants to be left alone.	Light. Noise. Movement and jarring. Hot rooms. Any effort or demand	Passing a lot of urine. Napping. Being left alone	Gelsemium
Migraines of sudden, violent onset with very flushed face	Intense, throbbing pains with oversensitivity to stimulation. Irritable, bad-tempered and feverish. Pains extend from the forehead to the back of the head. Bright red, hot and dry face, with cold hands and feet. Pains may go as abruptly as they began.	Light. Noise. Movement and jarring. In the afternoon. Stooping. Lying down	Firm pressure. Sitting up. Cool applied locally. Fresh air	Belladonna

TYPE	GENERAL INDICATIONS	WORSE FROM	BETTER FOR	REMEDY NAME
Migraines with terrific sensitivity to the slightest motion	Very irritable and bad-tempered with pain which is bursting and splitting. Pain may lodge in the forehead over the left eye. Terrible sensitivity to movement of any part of the body: even moving the eyes makes the pain worse. Migraine may be triggered by constipation.	Motion. Warmth. Eating. Constipation. Being disturbed	Cool in general. Cool air. Lying down. Firm pressure. Keeping completely still. Being left alone	Bryonia
Right-sided migraines that affect the right shoulder	Pains start at the back of the head and radiate to the right shoulder. Very sick, shivery and nauseated with migraine. Onset of attacks in morning which are better by the evening. Pains are sharp, splitting and cutting and are relieved by vomiting.	Jolting or jarring. Noise. In the morning	Sleep. Firm pressure. Vomiting. Onset of evening	Sanguinaria
Migraines that are made worse by vomiting	Periodic migraines, e.g. every weekend, that are preceded by blurred vision. Scalp feels tight and there may be increased flow of saliva with pain. Attack may be brought on by eating too many sweet things.	Vomiting. Sweet foods. Constipation	Walking in the open air	Iris

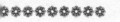

TYPE	GENERAL INDICATIONS	WORSE FROM	BETTER FOR	REMEDY NAME
Left-sided migraines that briefly feel better for cool bathing: then worse	Stiff neck and shoulders with migraine. Eye sockets may also feel very sensitive. Left eye waters during pain. Hypersensitive to pain with possible palpitations. Numb feeling at nape of the neck with sensitive back of the head.	Movement. Stooping. After washing with cold water. Noise	Warmth. Lying with head raised	Spigelia
Migraines that are brought on by eating too many rich, fatty foods	Pains may be located in forehead but change their location frequently. Migraines may come on before, during or after period had ended. Nausea and vomiting accompany pains. May be irritable and weepy but feel much better for sympathy and attention. Adversely affected by becoming warm.	Stuffy rooms. Warmth in general. Rest. At night. Blowing the nose	Fresh, open air. Gentle motion in the open air. Sympathy. Attention. Cool in any form. Firm pressure	Pulsatilla
Migraines that are relieved by vigorous exercise	One-sided migraines with shooting pains and marked sensitivity to cooking smells and perfume which makes nausea worse. Very irritable, depressed and tearful with pain: cannot tolerate demands of family life.	Light. Noise. Strong odours. Emotional demands. Before a period. Thundery weather	Sleep. Vigorous exercise, especially out of doors. Firm pressure. Warm bed	Sepia

Seek professional advice:

- If you experience a headache following a fall.

- If your symptoms are more severe than usual or last longer than you would expect.

- If you experience slurring of speech, numbness, dizziness or weakness of one side of your body accompanied by head pain for the first time, or if the usual pattern of these symptoms has changed.

- If you develop a migraine after beginning the contraceptive pill or any new medication.

- If you consistently have a headache on waking, or persistent headaches.

CHAPTER 5

PREGNANCY AND CHILDBIRTH

The experience of pregnancy and childbirth can be one of the most exciting and rewarding events that we encounter in our lives. However, as with any challenging and demanding situation, this can be a time when things just feel 'too much' and exhaustion sets in. For this reason, it is essential to use any practical advice available in order to enhance our overall health before conception, during pregnancy, and after childbirth. This is especially true for mothers who start their families in their thirties or early forties, who need to conserve energy levels as much as possible in order to deal with sleepless nights and busy days.

Within this context, homoeopathic treatment has an enormous amount to offer because it is a system of healing that is designed to stimulate and boost the body's capacity for self-healing and energy production. Unlike many orthodox drugs which cannot be taken during pregnancy (especially for the first three months), homoeopathic medicines are frequently administered to expectant mothers and have never been known to cause untoward side-effects.

If problems are persistent, or refuse to respond to self-help measures, it is vitally important to seek professional help. You will find that many of the conditions mentioned below will be substantially improved by general changes in diet or

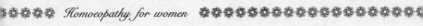

lifestyle, and do not require any extra help from homoeopathic medicines.

For advice on how to use the remedy tables, please see the section entitled **Using this book: Selecting the right remedy** on page 19. To obtain the best results it is essential to read this information first and follow the directions as closely as possible, rather than attempting to use the tables without instructions.

Morning sickness

There are many straightforward ways of helping to ease or banish the misery of morning sickness and nausea in early pregnancy. Although this usually occurs in the first three months it can last much longer in some cases. The term 'morning sickness' can also be rather misleading since some women find they feel nauseated and vomit only in the mornings, but others find they are sick any time of day or evening.

Basic self-help measures

• Eat small amounts frequently, even if nausea is present. Nausea and morning sickness can be made much worse by low or unstable blood sugar levels, therefore it is essential to eat small amounts of easily digested foods regularly in order to stabilise blood sugar as much as possible. Choose light, digestible foods, such as fruit, soups, or low fat sources of protein, such as fish or chicken. Avoid heavy, indigestible forms of protein, such as full fat cheese or greasy meat, highly flavoured snack foods such as crisps, or sugary convenience foods and drinks.

• Although the foods recommended above give a rough idea of the ideal foods to eat, remember that you should also listen to your own body and eat whatever is appealing to you when you feel queasy.

• Experiment with eliminating certain food groups that you suspect may be making you feel worse. If these include dairy foods ensure that you are having enough calcium: green leafy vegetables such as broccoli and spinach, wholemeal bread and almonds are a good non-dairy source of this essential mineral. Also ensure you are having enough iron from nuts, seeds, eggs and pulses if you are not eating meat.

• When you wake, do not get up with an empty stomach, but eat something very light with a drink while you are in bed. A warm drink with dry toast or a biscuit would be ideal. Get up very slowly after you have finished and try to avoid moving around too quickly or stooping, especially if you feel dizzy.

• Avoid tea and coffee as much as possible (many women find they instinctively cannot abide the tastes of these beverages in pregnancy as the thought of the taste or smell makes them feel sick). Opt instead for herbal teas that soothe the digestion, such as peppermint or chamomile, or if coffee still appeals, consider switching to a barley or fig-based substitute that can be bought in powder or granule form.

• Try to relax as much as possible when eating and chew food very thoroughly: bolting food down will make you feel even more nauseated and uncomfortable.

• Morning sickness can be associated with feelings of ambivalence, confusion, and sometimes fear about being pregnant. These emotions can arise out of the blue in the early stages of pregnancy and cause a great deal of distress if kept bottled up, especially if this leads to additional feelings of guilt. If you suspect this may be the case, talk it over with anyone you feel close to, or someone with whom you feel at ease. This may be your partner, sister, mother, best friend, alternative health practitioner or GP. Remember that, however surprising and unexpected these emotions seem to be, they are experienced by many women during pregnancy and are nothing to be ashamed of.

Conventional treatment

Many GPs will stress the advice given above and try as far as possible to avoid giving drugs to control vomiting, especially during the first three months of pregnancy. However, if nausea and vomiting are persistent or severe, an antihistamine or an anti-emetic, such as metoclopramide, may be prescribed.

Homoeopathic treatment

If the self-help measures suggested above are effective, there may be no need for homoeopathic prescribing. However, if symptoms of morning sickness are still present, you may find an occasional dose of the appropriate homoeopathic remedy for your symptoms will give speedy and effective relief. If your symptoms are severe or if you do not respond to a

homoeopathic medicine which appears to fit your symptoms
always seek professional advice. Also seek help from a
homoeopathic practitioner if you find that you are needing to
take a remedy on more than a short-term basis to obtain
relief. Do remember that homoeopathic medicines are not
intended to be given on a daily basis for an extended period
of time.

TYPE	GENERAL INDICATIONS	WORSE FROM	BETTER FOR	REMEDY NAME
Morning sickness which is much worse in the mornings	Symptoms are relieved temporarily by eating, but quickly return. Terrible sensitivity to cooking smells. Very depressed, morose and bad-tempered. Ambivalent about being pregnant. Craves sour foods when hungry. Empty feeling in stomach accompanied by headache.	Skipping meals. Strong smells. Mornings. Cold. Emotional strain. Thinking about food	Eating	Sepia
Dreadful nausea that is not relieved by vomiting	Nausea is terribly distressing and made much worse by movement. Hot or cold sweat with feeling sick. Symptoms not improved by eating. Great difficulty in vomiting with empty belching and lots of saliva. Looks deathly pale.	Bending down. Movement. Eating. Vomiting. Smell of food. Cigarette smoke	Resting. Fresh air	Ipecac

TYPE	GENERAL INDICATIONS	WORSE FROM	BETTER FOR	REMEDY NAME
Frequent vomiting with chilliness and exhaustion	Faint and exhausted after vomiting. Vomits as soon as any food is eaten: much worse after cold food or drinks. Wants to be kept very warm with access to fresh air if headache is present. Terribly anxious and restless with vomiting. Mother generally anxious about her own state of health or that of her baby.	Cold. After eating or drinking. Movement. Being alone	Warmth. Sips of warm drinks. Keeping warm in bed. Lying down	Arsenicum album
Morning sickness which is worse in stuffy, airless rooms	Symptoms are aggravated by eating rich, creamy or fried foods. Nausea may be worse in the evening or at night and accompanied by weepiness. Although generally chilly, warmth in any form makes things worse.	At night or evenings. Stuffy rooms. Rich food. Being too warm in bed	Sympathy and attention. Cool, fresh air. Gentle movement out of doors. Having a good cry	Pulsatilla
Morning sickness with craving for salty foods	Withdrawn, sad and depressed with inability to talk over worries or anxieties about pregnancy. Aversion to, or craving for, bread, slimy foods or fat with marked thirst. Headaches may accompany morning sickness.	Sympathy and attention. Direct sunlight. Emotional release. Noise. Touch	Open air. Rest. Skipping meals. Being alone	Natrum mur

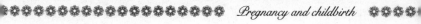

If morning sickness is persistent or severe, professional help should be sought.

Indigestion and Heartburn

It is very common for symptoms of indigestion and heartburn to occur in the middle or later stages of pregnancy. If these are mild and not causing distress, all that may be necessary are a few straightforward dietary adjustments and self-help measures to give the necessary relief.

Basic self-help measures

• Eat little and often, avoiding large meals after going for long periods without eating, especially late at night.

• Choose foods that are light, palatable and easy to digest. These include most vegetables, fruit, poultry, fish, and rice. If raw vegetables and fruit cause a problem, steam them lightly before eating to make them more easily digestible.

• Avoid foods that have a reputation for causing or aggravating indigestion. These include greasy, fried foods, hard full fat cheeses, raw onions and peppers, beans, pulses, citrus fruit, cabbage and tomatoes.

• If you enjoy cereal in the form of muesli but find it is very difficult to digest, try soaking it overnight in milk, fruit juice or water. This will partly break down the starch into sugar before you eat it. Other possibil-

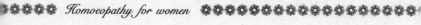

ities include switching to a cooked cereal, such as porridge.

• Avoid spicy foods, caffeine, alcohol and smoking as these all irritate the stomach lining. The last three should also be avoided in pregnancy since they may contribute to low birth weight and growth problems in babies.

• Eat slowly, chewing each mouthful thoroughly and try to avoid bolting, or grabbing food on the run.

• Switch to herbal teas (if you are not using homoeo-pathic medicines), such as peppermint, chamomile, or one of the many fruit blends available. Remember that it is a good idea to enjoy a range of teas rather than always drinking the same herbal variety. If you are taking homoeopathic medicines it is best to avoid peppermint in any form. This is because it is one of the substances that may interfere with the medicinal action of a homoeopathic remedy.

• If symptoms are troublesome at night, you may feel more comfortable sleeping propped up on a couple of extra pillows. However, this is contraindicated if you suffer from swollen ankles.

Conventional treatment

Your GP is likely to give general dietary advice about foods that aggravate indigestion and heartburn and may suggest the use of antacids to provide temporary relief of symptoms. Unfortunately, the latter are often aluminium-based preparations which can contribute to constipation. Sodium-based preparations, such as bicarbonate of soda,

should also be avoided since these can have an adverse effect on blood pressure.

Homoeopathic treatment

Homoeopathy has an excellent role to play in providing effective relief from the distressing symptoms of indigestion and heartburn. If these are only troublesome in the later stages of your pregnancy and you find that the occasional dose of your indicated remedy chosen from the table below gives speedy and effective relief, this may be all the help you need. However, if digestive problems are more of a long-term nature, or if they do not respond to self-help measures or the homoeopathic medicine you select, it is advisable to seek professional help.

TYPE	GENERAL INDICATIONS	WORSE FROM	BETTER FOR	REMEDY NAME
Indigestion with nausea and headache	Sensation of a hangover: headache, nausea, constipation and generally feeling 'out of sorts'. Headache is located across the eyes or at the back of the head. Lots of burping with a sour taste. Very irritable, bad-tempered and cold-sensitive.	Making any effort. Being deprived of sleep. On waking. Cold draughts. Stimulants	Rest. Napping. As the day goes on. Warmth	Nux vomica

TYPE	GENERAL INDICATIONS	WORSE FROM	BETTER FOR	REMEDY NAME
Acid indigestion with burning that is relieved by warm drinks	Chilliness with acidity and nausea. Heartburn aggravated by feeling anxious. Exhausted but cannot settle due to restlessness. Terrible burning in the stomach that is relieved by frequent sips of water or tea. Bouts of diarrhoea after eating fruit.	Any exertion. Cold in any form. At night. When alone	Sips of drinks at frequent intervals. Resting propped-up in bed. Warmth in any form. Company	Arsenicum album
Indigestion with excess wind and bloated sensation	Uncomfortable and distended after eating the slightest thing. Heavy and full sensations in stomach with frequent, violent burping. Has to loosen clothing constantly to be comfortable.	Stuffy rooms. Pressure of clothes. Warmth in general	Fresh, open air. Passing wind	Carbo veg
Indigestion with burping and noisy gurgling	Burning sensation extends from stomach to throat, when burping brings up a little acid each time. Even eating very little makes the stomach feel uncomfortably full. Feels worse from cold food and drinks and better from warm.	Eating a large meal. Tight clothes. In the afternoons. Cold food or drinks. Anxiety	Warmth. Loosening clothes. Open air. Being occupied. Warm food and drinks	Lycopodium

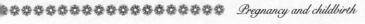

TYPE	GENERAL INDICATIONS	WORSE FROM	BETTER FOR	REMEDY NAME
Indigestion and heartburn which is aggravated by rich, fatty foods	Symptoms follow on from eating indigestible foods such as red meat, cheese, or creamy cakes or sauces. Dry mouth with no thirst and taste of food eaten hours before. Very weepy and subject to mood swings in pregnancy. Very sensitive to stuffy rooms and being over-heated.	Resting. Warmth. Stuffy rooms. Evening and night. Feeling neglected. Warm food or drinks	Open, fresh air. Gentle movement out of doors. Cool in any form. Sympathy and attention	Pulsatilla

If symptoms are severe, persistent and do not respond to self-help measures you should seek professional help.

Constipation

Many women who do not normally suffer from the misery of constipation are dismayed to find that they begin to suffer symptoms at some stage of their pregnancy. The reason for this is that the hormone progesterone, which maintains the condition of pregnancy, also adversely affects the tone of the bowel muscles, making them less likely to assist in achieving a regular or easy bowel movement. The growing foetus also tends to press on the large intestine, which also hinders the efficient working of the bowel. As a result, many of us suffer the unpleasant effects of constipation, which can include headaches, pain and discomfort, nausea, and generally feeling lethargic. This can be especially frustrating in the later stages of pregnancy, when energy levels may already be flagging. On the other hand, there are many simple steps we can take to remedy the situation.

Basic self-help measures

• First of all, look at the water content of your diet. It is easy to forget the importance of drinking enough water: ideally four or five large glasses each day. Remember that tea and coffee are not substitutes since they are diuretics: in other words, they encourage the body to rid itself of liquid instead of providing lubrication. Having an adequate intake of water also benefits the kidneys and helps discourage cystitis.

• Make sure you include large quantities of fresh fruit and vegetables in your diet to ensure that you are having enough fibre. An easy way to do this is to have a large salad with one main meal and fruit for dessert, and a large portion of fresh vegetables with the second main meal of the day and more fruit to follow. If you enjoy raw vegetables and find they do not cause indigestion, this is an excellent way of ensuring that you minimise the destruction of essential vitamins through cooking. However, if you prefer vegetables cooked, steam them lightly to preserve their crispness and vitamin content.

• If you do not suffer from digestive problems such as flatulence you can also increase the fibre content of your diet through including grains and pulses such as beans and lentils. When grains and pulses are combined in one meal they provide an excellent form of first-class protein. However, make sure you cook these ingre-

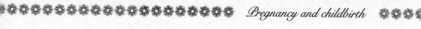

dients for the full time after soaking them beforehand, and take special care with beans, particularly red kidney beans, which must be thoroughly cooked before serving.

• Avoid foods which encourage constipation, such as dairy foods and fats. Ideally no more than twenty per cent of your total dietary intake should be made up of fat in any form. This includes cooking oils, eggs, cream, milk, cheese and meat. Also reduce foods which include refined products, such as white sugar and flour, especially where these are combined in one food, for instance cakes and biscuits. Introduce foods instead that use wholemeal, unrefined ingredients.

• Avoid cooking with aluminium pans or using tea bags which employ aluminium in their manufacturing process. Traces of aluminium in the diet are believed to aggravate a host of problems, including constipation and osteoporosis.

• Never put off the urge to pass a stool where possible, since this can encourage a problem to develop.

• Do not resort to laxatives in an effort to resolve the problem. Apart from the usual difficulties associated with their use, such as a tendency to become dependent on them to achieve a bowel movement, there is also a risk of miscarriage or premature labour following laxative use in pregnancy. General problems also associated with protracted laxative use include a cycle of alternating constipation and diarrhoea. This can eventually lead to a state of malabsorption where essential nutrients are not given a chance to be utilised by the body.

Conventional treatment

If dietary advice does not solve the problem, a non-oily laxative may be prescribed.

Homoeopathic treatment

An appropriately selected homoeopathic medicine can be immensely helpful in encouraging the body to deal with an acute bout of constipation, especially if this is linked to a day or two of overindulgence or eating unwisely. If, on the other hand, constipation is becoming an on-going feature of your pregnancy and the basic advice given above has not resolved the situation, or you have not responded to the homoeopathic medicine that fits your symptoms most closely, help should be sought from a homoeopathic practitioner. This is especially important if you have an underlying tendency to constipation and have a history of relying on medication to keep the situation stable.

TYPE	GENERAL INDICATIONS	WORSE FROM	BETTER FOR	REMEDY NAME
Constipation with no urge to pass a stool	Irritability, nausea and headache with constipation. Listless and averse to moving around. Feeling of inactivity in bowel: unaware of any need to pass a stool. Stool is dry, hard and very large. Intense thirst for cold drinks.	Any effort. Warmth. Being disturbed. Moving around	Keeping still. Cold drinks. Cool in general	Bryonia

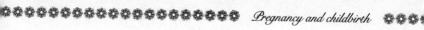

TYPE	GENERAL INDICATIONS	WORSE FROM	BETTER FOR	REMEDY NAME
Constipation brought on by change of routine or anxiety	Lots of urging and straining which doesn't achieve anything. Bloating of abdomen with rumbling, gurgling noises and frequent passage of wind. May feel very anxious about being constipated.	Eating. Anything tight around waist or abdomen. Becoming tired. When travelling or out of routine	Warm drinks. Undoing clothes	Lycopodium
Constant urging and straining with constipation: feeling of never quite having finished	Bad-tempered and headachey with constipation. Problem of 'bashful stool': feels as though bowel movement has been incomplete. Grouchy and cold-sensitive: always feels worse if exposed to cold draughts. Often indicated after painkillers, stimulants, or general overindulgence.	Being disturbed. Broken sleep. Eating. Stimulants. Getting cold	Resting. Being left alone. Undisturbed sleep	Nux vomica

TYPE	GENERAL INDICATIONS	WORSE FROM	BETTER FOR	REMEDY NAME
Soft, sticky stool with constipation	Itching and burning of anus with constipation. Stool may be soft and sticky or hard and knotted: either way it is very difficult to pass. Bowel feels totally inactive. May be much worse from, or averse to, a starchy diet.	Sitting still. Alternate days. When feeling cold	Eating. Warm food and drinks. Warmth in general	Alumina
Constipation with tendency to anal fissure	Days go by without any possibility of a bowel movement. When it occurs, stool is like sheep dung (small balls or pellets) which may be covered in mucus. Once a motion is achieved, there may be aching and discomfort in rectum for a while.	Over-exertion. Getting overheated. Cold drinks. At night in bed	Resting. Being well wrapped-up and warm. Fresh air	Graphites

Seek professional advice if:

• stools are discoloured: especially if they are very dark, grey or white;

• you have not had a bowel movement for twenty-four hours and you are conscious of pain;

• stools are difficult to pass or if you experience alternating constipation and diarrhoea;

- there is any unexplainable change in your bowel movements or bleeding;

- you notice a yellow tinge to your skin or eyes.

High Blood Pressure

If this is a problem which extends beyond minor fluctuations in blood pressure readings and has become a persistent feature during pregnancy, it is a situation which should not be treated by self-help prescribing. Your GP or midwife will need to monitor your blood pressure readings carefully if they are on the high side, in order to check that other conditions which are related to elevated blood pressure do not set in.

When your blood pressure is taken, you will see that it is reflected in two sets of figures such as 120/80. The upper figure refers to the measurement taken when your heart is beating, and the lower one to the measurement when your heart is at rest. The former is called the systolic reading and the latter the diastolic. High blood pressure may be calculated as a reading of 130/90 or above, or may be based on an increase of 30 points above your normal systolic, and 15 points increase on your normal diastolic readings.

Basic self-help measures

- Be aware of the strong relationship between stress and raised blood pressure. Look objectively at your daily routine and see if there are any steps you can take to lift some stress off your shoulders. Sit down with a pen and paper and write down all of the stressful factors that are present in your life. Prioritise this list, working out what is absolutely essential, and what can be given a lower priority, omitted, or delegated to someone else. Also make a list of things which you find relaxing, pleasurable and refreshing and give these as much priority as possible in your daily routine. Most important of all, ensure that you spend some time on your own each day – your space in which to unwind and relax.

• Explore relaxation techniques or meditation and devote a regular time each day to using either. If you also learn how to breathe for relaxation from your diaphragm you can use this as a tool any time of day you are feeling stressed or overwrought. Consider going to a yoga class, since yoga teachers are especially good at teaching breathing techniques to induce relaxation. Yoga is also an excellent form of exercise in pregnancy, with its emphasis on encouraging muscular suppleness, strength and stamina.

• Be aware that certain situations can result in raised blood pressure readings. Having your blood pressure monitored after a long or frustrating wait in a hospital waiting room is likely to cause a rise in your reading. On the other hand, if you can have your blood pressure monitored at home by your midwife in familiar surroundings, the chances are that the result may be more representative of your average state.

• Make sensible dietary changes. Eliminate salt, tea, coffee and chocolate as much as possible from your diet. If you smoke, be aware that this will contribute in the long run to the problem, and that it is advantageous to cut down, or ideally, cut out cigarettes. Drink as much water as possible and introduce soothing caffeine-free herbal teas in moderation, such as chamomile. Also make sure that you have enough protein each day from sources such as fish, chicken, pulses and rice, and eat three or four good helpings each day of fresh fruit and vegetables.

• Ask for as much help as possible from friends and family in order to relieve some of the pressure. If emotional strain is great, consider additional help from counselling.

• Seek professional help from an alternative health practitioner.

If the following occur, seek medical help as soon as possible:

• Unexplained gain in weight, puffy ankles or wrists that do not go down overnight.

• Headaches.

• Nausea and vomiting.

• Blurred vision.

• Light-sensitivity.

Labour and Childbirth

Homoeopathic medicines can have a very positive role to play during labour in facilitating each stage and enabling the mother to cope with exhaustion and pain. Although difficult in such an emotionally charged situation, it is possible for a husband or partner to familiarise himself with the possible remedies that might be needed. This is ideally best done by having a joint session before the birth with mother, partner and homoeopath, where specific remedies can be discussed, along with their application in problem situations. Remember that on a practical level, it is necessary to have a consultant sufficiently interested in, or sympathetic towards alternative medicine to sanction the use of homoeopathic remedies during labour and delivery.

If this is the case, especially if you have the support of your midwife, it is worth asking your homoeopath if they would be willing to attend the birth. Increasing numbers of alternative practitioners are now offering their services in this capacity as small but increasing numbers are being introduced into the NHS system.

The following table lists just a few of the possible homoeopathic medicines that may be needed in the different stages of labour. The function of this table is to give you a rough idea of some of the possible remedies that can be helpful in labour.

TYPE	GENERAL INDICATIONS	WORSE FROM	BETTER FOR	REMEDY NAME
Labour slow to get underway with lots of changeable pains	Contractions begin but are slow to progress; they keep stopping and starting. Marked mood swings with tendency to weepiness and despondency. Much worse for a stuffy room: needs fresh air. Mothers needing Pulsatilla often have a baby in a posterior or breech position.	Warmth. Keeping still. Lack of attention	Cool, fresh air. Cool applications. Moving around. Comfort and sympathy	Pulsatilla

TYPE	GENERAL INDICATIONS	WORSE FROM	BETTER FOR	REMEDY NAME
Sharp labour pains that seem to fly in all directions but which don't accomplish anything	Contractions are long, slow, very painful and unfruitful. Sharp pains migrate to groin and bladder. Shivering with weak labour pains. Often needed if dilation of cervix has begun but then decreases, provided other symptoms agree. Wants fresh air, but feels cold-sensitive. Irritability with exhaustion and trembling.	Exhaustion. Exposure to cold	Fresh air	Caulophyllum
Terrible anxiety with onset of labour	Very restless with anxiety: convinced that something will go wrong and that she will die. Moves from fear of death to feeling she wants to die. Often indicated in short, violent, frightening labour.	Extremes of warmth or cold. Examina-tion or touch	Fresh air. Uncovering	Aconite

TYPE	GENERAL INDICATIONS	WORSE FROM	BETTER FOR	REMEDY NAME
Backache labour with anxiety and complete exhaustion	Very weary at beginning of labour: anticipates that she doesn't have the energy to go through with it. Contractions in the back with very heavy and weak feelings in legs. Very sensitive to being examined: contractions may stop.	Exhaustion. Anticipating labour	Sweating	Gelsemium
Backache labour that is relieved by firm pressure to back	Pains travel from small of back to buttocks. Relief is provided by massage or pressure to affected area. Lots of burping and flatulence with contractions. Squatting with elbows on knees speeds up contractions. Irritable and bossy during labour.	Becoming cold. Uncovering	Warmth. Hard pressure	Kali carb

TYPE	GENERAL INDICATIONS	WORSE FROM	BETTER FOR	REMEDY NAME
Very irritable with straining sensations	Exhausted, weary and very irritable or abusive in labour. Mother constantly feels as though she needs to pass a stool when in pain. Backache labour with dragging, aching, bruised pains. Retching through labour with difficulty bringing up vomit.	Very cold-sensitive. Uncovering. Fresh air	Warmth	Nux vomica
Unbearable pain with terrific anger and irritability	Enraged by pains which mother feels she cannot tolerate any longer. Unfruitful labour pains which are felt in the back. Cervix dilates too slowly leaving mother furious and impatient. Face is either red or one side may be red and the other pale.	Fresh air	Uncovering. Sweating	Chamomilla

Homoeopathy after the birth

There is an enormous amount that can be done to ease the pain and distress following labour and delivery by using the appropriate homoeopathic remedy. The potential scope is very wide, with homoeopathic medicines being given internally and externally in the form of diluted tinctures, creams and lotions. The value of homoeopathic prescribing at this stage is immense, since the appropriate remedy will speed up healing, ease pain and guard against possible infection. The following table will give you a basic idea of the remedies you should consider after labour and delivery.

TYPE	GENERAL INDICATIONS	WORSE FROM	BETTER FOR	REMEDY NAME
Aching, bruised pains with extreme tenderness	The first remedy to give after delivery in order to speed up reabsorption of blood, ease pain of bruised tissue, and support the mother to deal with shock and trauma after childbirth. Difficulty finding comfortable position in bed.	Touch. Jarring. Being approached	Lying down	Arnica
Pain which follows an episiotomy or tear	Use this remedy in diluted tincture, cream or ointment form. Add the tincture to bath water, or saturate a sanitary pad with diluted tincture to keep it in contact with painful area. Cream or ointment can be applied after the lotion or diluted tincture.	Cold	Keeping still	Calendula

TYPE	GENERAL INDICATIONS	WORSE FROM	BETTER FOR	REMEDY NAME
Shooting pains from an incision or tear	Often indicated after forceps delivery, or where back pain follows epidural. Pains are tearing, shooting and bruised. Hypericum may be combined with Calendula to form Hypercal tincture.	Touch or contact of any kind. Moving		Hypericum
Stinging, sharp pains from stitches or after Caesarian section	Often needed after highly mechanised childbirth when expectations were different. Terrible feelings of anger, resentment, violation, or having been cheated.	Motion. Pressure	Warmth	Staphysagria
Deep bruising that has not been resolved by Arnica	Indicated where Arnica has helped with initial phase of bruising, but tenderness and sensitivity remain.	Touch. Warm bathing	Motion. Cool applied locally.	Bellis perennis

Post-natal Depression or 'Baby Blues'

The emotional fluctuations that follow pregnancy and childbirth can be extremely confusing, unpredictable and overwhelming. Many women have been amazed at the range of emotions they go through in the early weeks or months of getting to know their baby. These feelings can include anger, weepiness, euphoria, sadness, lack of confidence, loneliness, confusion and shock. If feeling depressed lasts for a protracted period of time, you may be suffering from post-natal depression. The symptoms are varied, but the following are representative of the condition in general:

- Low self-esteem.

- Anxious feelings, especially about your baby.

- Sleep disturbance, above and beyond what would normally be expected with looking after a young baby.

- Hopelessness or despair.

- Overwhelmed and unable to cope with day-to-day demands.

- Feeling flat, dazed, numb or distanced from things.

- Exhaustion that is not relieved by rest and relaxation.

Predisposing factors

- Women who lack the support of a caring and sympathetic partner, family or friends.

- Mature women who have been very career oriented, who react badly to the fundamental change in their circumstances that motherhood brings.

- Severe stress in pregnancy, such as bereavement, moving home, or giving up a satisfying job.

- Women who feel a sense of grief or sadness when their baby is born because of a sense of separation.

• Women who experience a painful, protracted labour with more medical intervention than they were prepared for; especially if birth was by an unplanned Caesarian section.

Basic self-help measures

• Acknowledge your feelings and do not be afraid to ask for help from friends, close relatives or a more formal source, such as a counsellor.

• Talk over your feelings as much as you need to, especially those feelings associated with the birth of your baby.

• Keep in contact with at least one new mother you may have met at relaxation classes. It is vital that you feel you have access to someone who will be exploring similar challenges, fears and doubts.

• Resist advice that suggests all you need is a stiff upper lip: acknowledge your emotions rather than feeling they will go away if they are ignored or repressed.

• If you are feeling remote or lonely, use the telephone to keep in contact with those you can talk to honestly and candidly.

• Arrange to have time away from your baby when you are free to do something unrelated to motherhood.

• If you feel tense and on edge most of the time, arrange to have a regular back or full body massage as often as you can.

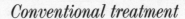

Conventional treatment

Depending on the duration and severity of the problem, possible options include antidepressants, tranquillisers, hormone therapy and psychiatric help.

Homoeopathic treatment

If you experience fleeting feelings of being 'down' after childbirth, one of the following remedies may help you over a temporary state of depression. However, if you feel that you are entering a more long-term depressive state, it is essential that you seek help from a homoeopathic or alternative health practitioner in order to help you over the condition. As with chronic (long-term) anxiety or depression, self-help prescribing is not appropriate within this context. On the other hand, 'baby blues' can be treated appropriately by a homoeopathic practitioner, with the advantage that the remedies prescribed do not have the attendant drawbacks associated with tranquillisers or hormone therapy.

TYPE	GENERAL INDICATIONS	WORSE FROM	BETTER FOR	REMEDY NAME
Weepiness or sadness after childbirth that is helped by sympathy	Very tearful and generally subject to mood swings. Responds well to attention and a sympathetic ear: feels relief after a good cry in the company of someone who cares. Often indicated soon after birth.	Feeling neglected. All attention focused on the baby. Being in stuffy, airless rooms all day. Lacking exercise	Sympathy and attention. Crying. Hugs and cuddles. Fresh, open air. Gentle exercise	Pulsatilla

TYPE	GENERAL INDICATIONS	WORSE FROM	BETTER FOR	REMEDY NAME
Very emotional and subject to contradictory moods in days after birth	Severe mood swings which alternate from spasmodic, involuntary weeping to euphoria in a very short space of time. Indicated where mother feels overwhelming sense of grief at being separated from her baby. Constant sighing with anxiety and excitability.	Stimulants such as coffee or tobacco. Alcohol. Getting chilled. Fresh air	Warmth. Eating. Being distracted by outside involvements	Ignatia
Apathetic and irritable with feeling of distance from baby	Physically and mentally exhausted and worn out. Often too little time between pregnancies. Lack of interest in anything including new baby, partner or sex. Reacts badly to physical affection, touch or sympathy. Much better for vigorous exercise.	Sympathy or attention. Any over-exertion. Resting. Going without meals. Being touched	Stimulation through exercise: aerobics, housework or running. Eating regularly. Fast walking. After a nap. Being warm in bed	Sepia

TYPE	GENERAL INDICATIONS	WORSE FROM	BETTER FOR	REMEDY NAME
Depression with strong desire to be alone	Although profoundly depressed, weeping does not come easily. If it does, mother feels much worse afterwards. Cannot stand sympathy, and rejects it when offered. Easily hurt and tends to repress feelings, especially grief. Cannot bear to be seen crying in public: feels humiliated.	Sympathy. Weeping. Attention. Physical effort. After eating	Being left alone. Resting	Nat mur
Anger, indignation and a sense of humiliation with depression	Often indicated after a 'high tech' birth or Caesarian where mother feels very angry and cheated at not giving birth the way she intended to. May feel violated as a result of invasive procedures. Indicated where pain from stitches is excruciating, or where pain has remained in old scars.	Touch. Pressure. Sexual contact. Mental effort	Resting. After eating. Warmth	Staphysagria

TYPE	GENERAL INDICATIONS	WORSE FROM	BETTER FOR	REMEDY NAME
Gloomy, depressed state with fear of hurting the baby	Talkative and agitated or very downcast with depression. Very afraid that something terrible is going to happen, or that she is about to go insane. Very fidgety, excitable and nervous. Sighs all the time when feeling down.	Cold. Damp conditions	Movement. Warmth. Open air	Cimicifuga

If any of the following problems occur, you must seek professional help:

- A sense of losing touch with reality or a sensation of separation from others, with attendant feelings of anger or emotional numbness.

- Constant feelings of anxiety or forebodings about things that would normally cause no problem.

- Depressive feelings that are severe or persistent and which do not respond to self-help measures.

Mastitis

Care and prompt action need to be taken if you suspect you have a blocked duct, in order to prevent the more severe condition of mastitis (breast abscess) developing. Initial indications include:

• Soreness and a lumpy feeling in the affected breast.

• There may, or may not be, redness affecting the skin above the lump.

• If a high temperature develops, this is an indication that you have a problem with mastitis and need to seek professional help.

Basic self-help measures

• Check that your bra is not too tight.

• Use a simple hydrotherapy technique by applying hot and cool flannels alternately to the affected breast. Start with a flannel which has been soaked in hot water and wrung out. Place this over the painful breast until it has cooled. Take the flannel off, and apply another that has been dipped in cool water for about five to ten minutes. Keep this process up for an hour or two.

• Breastfeed more frequently to ensure that you drain the milk from all of the ducts. Experiment with your baby in different positions in order to find which one enables him or her to feed most easily and efficiently.

• Use a breast pump if your breasts feel full as a result of your baby not wanting to feed regularly.

• Take in regular and increased amounts of fluid.

• Feed your baby from the affected side first, ensuring that this side is fully emptied at each feed.

• Use the force of gravity to help drain the blocked duct by positioning your breast and baby in such a way that the painful area is uppermost.

- When your baby is feeding, massage your breasts gently towards the nipple. You can also massage your breasts between feeds.

- If you have been doing too much and feel generally run down, ask for help and go to bed for a day or two. Bed rest at the early stage of a problem can prevent a more serious phase developing.

- Swing your arms regularly in order to encourage blood flow.

Conventional treatment

The possible options include antibiotics or draining the abscess. However, antibiotics are best avoided if you are breastfeeding.

Homoeopathic treatment

Prompt use of the most appropriate homoeopathic medicine in the early stage of a breast abscess can be enormously helpful in preventing the situation becoming more serious. Skilled use of homoeopathy at the first sign of inflammation can render the use of antibiotics unnecessary. This is a tremendous advantage for breastfeeding mothers who can continue to feed their babies while taking homoeopathic remedies, since this form of treatment will not have any adverse effects on their baby.

As it is vital that you choose the most appropriate remedy as quickly as possible, contact your homoeopath if you feel unsure of which of the following remedies to choose. Also get professional help if you develop any sign of a rise in temperature, or if you feel you are not responding to your selected remedy within twenty-four hours.

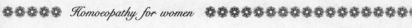

TYPE	GENERAL INDICATIONS	WORSE FROM	BETTER FOR	REMEDY NAME
Pain in breast which is very much worse for movement	Breast feels hard and painful and is much worse for even the slightest movement. Instinctively wants to press against the painful area. Irritable and intolerant of everyone: just wants to be left alone.	Slight movement. Jarring. Heat. Making any effort	Lying very still. Cool in general. Firm pressure. Lying on the painful side	Bryonia
Mastitis with shooting pains all over the body	Pains in breasts may shoot to armpit: glands generally may feel swollen and tender. Sore, cracked nipples and hard, swollen, stony purple-looking breasts. Very depressed, worn out and shivery with pains.	Damp and cold. Getting heated in bed. Touch. Lying on the right side. At night	Moderate warmth. Lying on the stomach or on the left side	Phytolacca
Violent onset of severe pain with extreme sensitivity to touch	Very dry, bright red, hot skin with red streaks running from nipple along breast. Very intolerant of being disturbed in any way: cannot stand noise, bright light or any form of stimulation. Lying down in bed makes pain worse.	The least jolt or jarring movement. Touch. Lying on affected side. Being disturbed	Lying semi-erect in bed. Being left in peace. Warmth	Belladonna

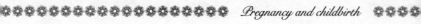
TYPE	GENERAL INDICATIONS	WORSE FROM	BETTER FOR	REMEDY NAME
General swelling and lumpiness of breasts made much worse by warmth	Pain comes in intense bouts that reduce mother to tears. Subject to severe mood swings with pains. Although chilly, feels much worse for warmth in any form. Although pressure helps, heavy bedclothes can aggravate the pain and discomfort.	Heat. Resting. Heavy clothes or bedclothes. In the evening or at night	Cool, fresh air. Gentle movement. Pressure. Sympathy and attention	Pulsatilla
Hard, swollen breasts with cracked, sore nipples	Exhausted and chilly with a strong desire to go to bed. Symptoms may be left-sided. Sleepless by night and drowsy by day with pain. Hot, flushed face with icy hands and feet. Fissures in nipples cause great distress.	Cold. Damp. Becoming overheated. At night. Lying on left side	Fresh air. Being warmly wrapped-up. Resting	Graphites
Terrible anxiety and restlessness with pains that feel much worse at night	Exhausted, sweaty and trembling with pains. Cannot get comfortable due to sensitivity to slightest variation in temperature. Tosses and turns all night with restlessness and pain.	Marked heat or cold. In bed. At night. Slightest draught. Touch or pressure. Sweating	Resting in moderate temperatures	Mercurius

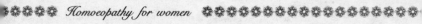

If self-help measures have not been successful within twenty-four hours, or if you show signs of feverishness, you must seek professional help.

CHAPTER 6

THE LATER YEARS: MENOPAUSE AND BEYOND

The years leading up to the menopause are often filled with fear, apprehension and uncertainty for the majority of women. Threats of loss of identity, fear of growing old, sorrow over children leaving home, and the physical changes that attend the menopause are all common areas of concern.

However, there is another side to the picture that is becoming increasingly apparent as women take a more positive stance in demanding further information about what we can realistically expect as we pass beyond the menopause. Popular writers such as Gail Sheehy have contributed enormously to this change of attitude by providing a new perspective to the years that constitute this radical change, and giving a realistic appraisal of the pros and cons associated with it.

By becoming better informed and more fully prepared for the changes that are ahead of us, it is possible to take a proactive stance. If we share our uncertainties, fears and insecurities with others who have gone through similar emotions, we may also experience the comfort and reassurance of knowing that we are not alone. Most important of all, we can discover that there is an end to the turbulence, after which we may be left feeling more empowered and clear-headed about our decision-making and meeting our needs than previously.

Within this context, holistic approaches to healing have a tremendous amount of offer. This is because they provide as much information and guidance as possible to enable the patient to elevate their experience of health and overall well-being. At this time of life, we must be especially aware of the importance of foods that will help us and those that do the opposite. We also need to explore the most appropriate forms of exercise and movement for our needs if we are to keep mobile and fit. By putting this information into practice, we have the best chance of looking forward to an active, positive experience of later life.

For advice on how to use the remedy tables, please see the section entitled **Using this book: Selecting the right remedy** on page 19. To obtain the best results it is essential to read this information first and follow the directions as closely as possible, rather than attempting to use the tables without instructions.

Hot Flushes

Hot flushes are the symptom most of us associate with the menopause, and they have traditionally been the trigger for a variety of reactions which range from panic to uneasy laughter. The severity, duration and time of onset of hot flushes can vary enormously from one woman to another, but there are certain characteristics that will be commonly shared by those who experience them. These include:

- A tendency to overheat or 'flush up' in situations where fresh air is in short supply, or surroundings are generally too warm. The onset can be extremely abrupt and violent, or we may experience a brief sense of foreboding before the flush begins. During a flush, our skin becomes suffused with blood and turns bright pink.

• Drenching sweats may accompany the flush. These can cover the face, neck, chest or whole body. These can be extremely distressing because of their severity, leaving us feeling soaking wet, clammy, and generally wrung-out.

• Hot flushes are often associated with sleep disturbance, with many of us waking a few seconds before a flush begins. These are called night sweats and may happen once or twice a night, or more frequently, leaving us shattered by morning.

• It is not uncommon for hot flushes to be accompanied by a sense of panic or extreme anxiety. This may be a generalised sensation, or a specific dread that someone will notice that we are having a hot flush.

• Fatigue, dizziness and headaches may also accompany hot flushes.

Basic self-help measures

• Learn how to breathe in order to induce relaxation and to minimise stress reactions. (See section on *Insomnia* in Chapter 2.) By learning these simple breathing techniques we have a tool that can be used any time we are under stress and feeling panicked. This has the benefit of helping us feel empowered and focused in a situation that can otherwise leave us feeling helpless and frightened.

• Explore meditation, visualisation and relaxation

techniques in order to help you re-evaluate your reactions to stress and clear your mind. Once you have found a technique that you are happy with, incorporate in into your daily routine. By doing so, you are ensuring that you spend some time each day on yourself.

• Guard against low blood sugar levels (hypoglycaemia) by eating small amounts regularly, and avoiding large gaps between meals. Also steer clear of foods that appear to play havoc with blood sugar levels. These include: strong tea, coffee, caffeinated fizzy drinks; foods that combine refined flour, fat and sugar, such as cakes, biscuits and chocolate. Concentrate instead on nutritious snacks such as crudités made from any crisp, raw vegetables in season that you enjoy; dips made from seasoned, live natural yoghurt, or fromage frais with chopped chives or spring onions; rice cakes with cheese or any other toppings that appeal, and fresh fruit in season. Be as imaginative as you need in making snacks that are exciting and tasty, but try to make sure that whatever you use is as fresh as possible, and close to its natural state rather than tinned or dehydrated. The symptoms of hypoglycaemia may include:

  • abrupt mood swings;
  • initial energy spurts after eating, followed by exhaustion;
  • fuzzy thinking, confusion and forgetfulness;
  • sleepiness following meals.

• Make time for regular, enjoyable exercise that is vigorous enough to produce a sweat. Good examples include: cycling, running, brisk walking uphill, dancing, or low-impact aerobics. In order to have maximum

beneficial impact, it is best to begin an exercise plan before menopausal symptoms have set in. Above all, make sure you choose a range of exercise that you enjoy in order to maintain enthusiasm and avoid boredom.

• If you have problems with insomnia as well as night sweats, avoid eating large meals late at night, stimulating caffeinated drinks, and above all, try to do something relaxing for a couple of hours before bedtime. (See section on *Insomnia* in Chapter 2 for additional suggestions.)

Conventional treatment

When menopausal symptoms, such as hot flushes, are severe, conventional doctors will often suggest Hormone Replacement Therapy (HRT) as a way of alleviating symptoms. The use of HRT has become an increasingly controversial issue, with a heated debate between those who disagree with its use and those who believe it is the most effective and beneficial way of dealing with menopausal symptoms. However, there appear to be definite contraindications to its use. These include anyone who has suffered from:

• chronic liver disease;
• cancer of the womb or breast.

Additional factors which might suggest an adverse reaction include:

• a history of endometriosis or fibroids;
• heart disease or circulatory problems;
• heavy smoking.

The main concern is that HRT may be implicated in an

increased risk of developing breast cancer during long-term use. Other problems associated with HRT include side-effects that many women are unable, or unwilling to tolerate. These may include headaches, depression, unacceptability of the return of period pains, and weight gain.

There are, in addition, broader areas of concern which have been fuelled by the popular press and television who have created the myth of HRT as an elixir of youth, prolonging our youthful looks and vitality well beyond middle age. For many of us, this has created an expectation that cannot be fulfilled, and which leads to bitter disappointment. It is also an attitude which does not help us prepare for, or ease into, our menopause with a realistic approach.

Problems that arise in the years following the menopause include an increased risk of heart disease (as oestrogen levels decrease) and osteoporosis (brittle bones). Those in favour of HRT believe that it helps protect against the development of these conditions, especially in those of us who have experienced an early menopause. Although we should be well into the menopause by the time we are fifty, many younger women will experience symptoms much earlier, some in the natural course of events, and others as a result of surgical intervention. For those of us who develop menopausal symptoms early, it is essential that we look to alternative measures for guarding against heart disease and osteoporosis if we choose to avoid HRT. It is also important to stress that HRT is still a very controversial area, with the final verdict being far from available with regard to its long-term effects.

For a more detailed account of the pros and cons of HRT, see the *Further Reading* section.

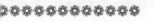

Homoeopathic treatment

If you are not severely troubled by hot flushes, but experience the odd minor flush on an irregular basis, an occasional dose of your appropriate remedy may help you over the problem. However, do remember that if you find you need to use your remedy on an increasingly frequent or regular basis to maintain an improvement, or if you find your symptoms are increasing in severity, it is essential to seek professional help rather than continuing to manage the situation by yourself. This is especially true if you have hot flushes within the broader context of other troublesome menopausal symptoms.

TYPE	GENERAL INDICATIONS	WORSE FROM	BETTER FOR	REMEDY NAME
Flushes which occur on first waking from sleep	Waves of heat through body, with cold feet. Hot flushes during the day, cold and clammy at night. Very talkative and inclined to be angry and jealous. Much worse for any constricting clothes, especially around the neck. Strong aversion to heat in any form.	Heat. Warm drinks. At night. On waking. Touch	Cool, fresh air. Cool drinks. Onset of a discharge. Eating a little. Gentle movement	Lachesis

TYPE	GENERAL INDICATIONS	WORSE FROM	BETTER FOR	REMEDY NAME
Violent flushes of heat with very dry skin	Flushes come on abruptly and severely with no warning. Skin becomes rapidly bright red, dry, and so uncomfortable that it radiates heat. Bouts of flushing end as rapidly as they began. Although head is burning, feet and hands feel icy cold. If sweats occur they feel boiling hot.	Jarring. Being chilled. Stimulation of any kind. Touch	Resting. Moderate warmth. Keeping still. Bending head back	Belladonna
Severe flushes that move upwards from chest to head	Pulsating hot flushes that come on very quickly. Disorientation, panic and palpitations with flushes. Sense of pressure in head with nausea and dizziness. Can't bear any sensation of heat about the head or sudden movement.	Heat. Movement. Extreme heat or cold. Humidity. Alcohol. Bending head back	Cool air, especially about head. Keeping very still	Glonoine
Localised flushes in face and neck	Circular, red patches on cheeks over area of cheek-bones. Patchy burning sensations on palms of hands, ears and soles of feet. Feels as though waves of heat are moving from one part of the body to another. Recurring right-sided headaches.	Cold. Humidity. Draughts. Touch. Exertion. At night	Sleep. Resting in the dark	Sanguinaria

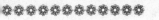
TYPE	GENERAL INDICATIONS	WORSE FROM	BETTER FOR	REMEDY NAME
Faintness and dizziness with hot flushes in stuffy rooms	Very sensitive to airless surroundings with a tendency to feel sick and faint before or during a flush. Very emotional and tearful with flushes, with marked improvement from sympathy. Too hot at night to get to sleep, or wakes from sleep in early hours of morning. Heavy night sweats.	Warm, airless rooms. Being too warmly dressed. Humidity. Heavy bed covers. Resting. At night or in evenings	Fresh, open air. Cool drinks or cool foods. Gentle exercise in the fresh air. Cool applied locally. Taking off or loosening clothes	Pulsatilla
Constant feeling of warmth with marked intolerance of heat	Although sensitive to heat, exposure to cold also causes discomfort. Easily exhausted with flushes of heat which are worse from standing or making physical effort: just wants to lie down in order to recover. Very uncomfortable in warm bed: pushes feet out of bed covers to cool them down.	Heat. Warmth of bed. Damp, cold. Bathing. Stimulation. After waking	Moderate temperatures. Lying down	Sulphur

If hot flushes are severe, persistent, or do not respond to self-help measures, professional help should be sought.

Stress Incontinence and Prolapse

Problems with incontinence and/or a prolapsed womb frequently occur after childbirth, especially if we have had two or more pregnancies close together, or if a labour has been lengthy and traumatic. The problems associated with these conditions can become more severe during or after the menopause as the uterine ligaments which hold up the womb tend to lose tone, and sag with increasing age. As with any condition, severity of symptoms can vary enormously, with some of us experiencing minor discomfort, inconvenience and embarrassment, and others in great distress with their quality of life being seriously affected. While there will be the variations outlined above, common symptoms can be identified. These include:

- Dragging sensations in the lower abdomen.

- Persistent backache.

- Difficulty emptying bladder and bowels, or a constant feeling as though needing to pass water.

- Small quantities of urine being passed involuntarily when exercising, coughing, laughing or sneezing.

- If prolapse is severe, a section of the vagina or uterus may protrude from the vaginal opening, resulting in soreness and irritation.

Basic self-help measures

- Exercise the muscles of the pelvic floor regularly by stopping and starting the flow of urine when you pass water. You may also exercise the whole of the pelvic floor if you concentrate on tightening as much of the vagina as possible.

• Rest as much as possible with your feet higher than your body, and avoid standing for long periods of time where possible.

• While gentle, regular exercise is generally beneficial, avoid any activities that are very vigorous or involve pounding, jarring movements, such as jogging.

• If you are overweight, lose the necessary amount by making sensible adjustments to your daily intake of food rather than crash dieting. Constructive measures include cutting out cakes, biscuits, alcohol (especially spirits that are combined with fizzy, sugar-laden mixers, such as tonic water), chocolates, and crisps. Eat at least two large helpings of raw, steamed vegetables and salad each day, and make sure you increase your intake of fresh fruit. Choose low fat forms of protein such as fish (unbattered and grilled), or chicken (discarding the skin), and eat large helpings of complex carbohydrates such as brown rice and pasta, adding sauces such as a strong-flavoured tomato and basil rather than using creamy or cheesy ingredients. Eat regular meals as far as possible and cut out snack foods. Also make sure that you do not eat a large meal before going to bed. This often leads to indigestion and heartburn, and encourages weight gain. The latter occurs because food eaten before sleep is not used as efficiently to provide energy at night as it is when we are active during the day. As a result, any excess calories taken in which are not utilised for energy production will be laid down as fat reserves.

Conventional treatment

For older women who have a mild prolapse, or where surgery is contraindicated, a ring pessary may provide sufficient support for short-term use. If the prolapse is severe, surgery may be indicated. This could involve a prolapse repair or a hysterectomy, depending on the degree of sagging involving the womb and cervix. Where stress incontinence is severe, surgery may be offered to strengthen the muscles of the pelvic floor.

Homoeopathic treatment

Where symptoms are mild and occasional, use of one of the following homoeopathic remedies may be very helpful, provided the symptoms agree. However, if stress incontinence is becoming an increasingly severe problem, or if the symptoms of prolapse are deteriorating, it is essential to seek professional help.

TYPE	GENERAL INDICATIONS	WORSE FROM	BETTER FOR	REMEDY NAME
Prolapse with exhaustion and backache	Onset of problem may date back to childbirth, but symptoms become most troublesome during menopause. Decrease in libido due to exhaustion and indifference to everything, including sexual partner. Constant bearing-down sensations with stream of urine slow to start.	Standing. Walking	Sitting with legs crossed. Warmth. Firm pressure	Sepia

TYPE	GENERAL INDICATIONS	WORSE FROM	BETTER FOR	REMEDY NAME
Marked incontinence on laughing, coughing, or sneezing	Discomfort greater when at rest, lying down or walking. Tearful, depressed and in need of sympathy with symptoms. Bladder symptoms may originate from pregnancy. Although chilly, craves fresh air.	At night. Resting. Becoming overheated	Cool, fresh air. Pressure. Sympathy. Weeping	Pulsatilla
General lack of muscle tone with vague aches and pains	Lethargy and general weakness with symptoms. Heavy feelings in uterus with constricted sensations, as though it were being squeezed by a band. Overwhelming need to lie down with a disinclination to make any kind of effort.	Hot rooms. Cold draughts. Making any effort	Fresh air. Stimulants. Passing large quantities of urine	Gelsemium
Prolapse with painful dryness of vagina	Introverted, depressed and withdrawn with menopausal symptoms. Aversion to love-making from dryness and pain in vagina. Urine may be slow to start, and may be passed involuntarily when walking or coughing. Low back pain that feels better for support in small of back.	Physical exertion. Walking. After sleep. Lying down	Open air. Gentle movement. Sitting with one leg crossed over the other. Pressure to mid back	Natrum mur

TYPE	GENERAL INDICATIONS	WORSE FROM	BETTER FOR	REMEDY NAME
Unconscious passage of large quantities of urine	Urine may escape suddenly when coughing or sneezing with no knowledge until after the event. Involuntary passing of urine at night, especially during early part of sleep. Incontinence develops slowly and progressively. General muscular weakness with strong desire to lie down.	Dry, cold weather. Draughts. Getting wet. After bathing. Travelling. Coffee	Warmth. Being warm in bed	Causticum

If symptoms are severe, persistent, or deteriorating, professional help should be sought.

Osteoporosis

This is a condition which has attracted a great deal of attention, especially with regard to the use of HRT as a way of protecting against calcium leaching out of the bones of those of us who are post-menopausal. The unfortunate result of calcium loss from our bones involves the risk of easy fractures, with particular risks being associated with trauma sustained by the neck of the femur (thigh bone). HRT (offering a combination of oestrogen and progesterone) has been hailed as the most effective way of preventing calcium loss from our bones. However, it must be stressed that accelerated bone loss occurs after the menopause for roughly fifteen years, and that HRT would have to be taken for a minimum of five years before there would be any noticeable reduction in the risk of fractures. This clearly involves a very long-term approach to drug therapy that many of us may feel uneasy about. Symptoms of osteoporosis include:

- Weakness of the pelvic floor.

- Restricted movement in the spine and chest.

- Well-established problems can be identified by the characteristic 'dowager's hump': this is the stooped appearance that many elderly women develop as they get older.

- Severe attacks of back pain or pain in weight-bearing joints.

- Loss of height.

- Muscle spasms and spontaneous fractures.

Predisposing factors

There are a number of factors which indicate that some women are more at risk than others with regard to developing osteoporosis. These include:

- Severe weight loss during adolescence, especially if combined with eating disorders.

- Use of steroids.

- Regular smoking or drinking alcohol.

- Lack of exercise which uses the weight-bearing joints.

- Poor quality or restricted diet.

• Conditions that involve difficulties in absorbing nutrients from food: bulimics are especially at risk.

Basic self-help measures

• Look to the quality of your diet, especially with regard to the amount of calcium taken on a daily basis. It is wise to do this as early as possible, rather than waiting until the menopause has begun in order to prevent bone mass being lost. Foods that are rich in calcium include: dairy products, such as cheese and milk, tofu, sardines, salmon (including the bones), and broccoli. Remember that not all calcium that is eaten is utilised by the body, and that this ability for absorption decreases as we get older. The following factors can adversely affect our ability to absorb calcium:

• Lack of exercise.

• Severe periods of stress or illness, especially if our periods stop.

• Eating large quantities of carbonated drinks, refined foods with processed ingredients.

• Too much animal protein in the diet.

If you feel you need to supplement the amount of calcium in your diet, remember that you must also supplement magnesium in order to utilise the calcium most effectively. The RDA (recommended daily allowance) for those of us who are pre-menopausal is 1000mg. Once we have reached the menopause, the RDA increases to 1,500mg.

• Keep as physically active as possible well before the menopause sets in. The best forms of exercise which

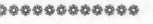

protect bone mass are those which involve vigorous movement of the weight-bearing joints. Choose from brisk walking, running, cycling or swimming, making sure that you enjoy whatever you do. You should aim for a minimum of three sessions per week, lasting thirty to forty-five minutes. This form of exercising has the additional benefit of conditioning your heart and circulatory system at the same time.

• Drink alcohol in moderation and make sure you have alcohol-free weeks or months. Drink as much filtered or spring water as possible, and avoid tap water containing fluoride. Also be aware that caffeinated drinks and smoking increase the leaching out of minerals from the bones.

• Consider supplementing with vitamins C, D (if you do not spend much time out of doors) and E if you suspect they are lacking in your diet.

Conventional treatment

The conventional approach in dealing with osteoporosis is to prescribe HRT for the reasons mentioned above. Additional dietary advice may also be given.

Homoeopathic treatment

Osteoporosis is a condition that should be dealt with in a professional context by a trained homoeopath who will look at your symptoms in the context of your overall health. Because of the long-term nature of the condition, and the often ill-defined nature of the symptoms, self-help prescribing is not appropriate. However, the self-help suggestions given above will be helpful as basic background measures.

It is possible for the appropriate homoeopathic medicine to have a positive effect on the quality of the skeletal system, provided you are being prescribed for as a whole person. Developing the skill of selecting a homoeopathic medicine which covers all symptoms presented by a patient requires professional expertise, knowledge of case analysis, and a thorough understanding of detailed information relating to each homoeopathic medicine. As you can imagine, this is something best left in the hands of an experienced practitioner.

'Empty Nest Syndrome'

This is a condition that springs out of a sense of loss, often occurring at a time when children are becoming independent and leaving home to make lives for themselves. If we chose to have children during our twenties and early thirties, they leave home when we are approaching or entering the menopause. If we have devoted our lives to homemaking and bringing up our children, this can be a time of great disruption and confusion, often leaving us with the feeling that we have become redundant. Even if we have a satisfying career, we may still not be exempt from feelings of distress at the prospect of the challenges we face moving on to middle age and beyond.

Additional demands that may be made on us during this time include the responsibility of caring for an ageing parent or other relative, which in turn will bring home to us that we are ageing ourselves. This is a situation that can give rise to a range of conflicting emotions including panic, fear, depression and a feeling that nothing is worth striving for.

 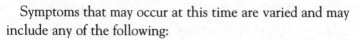

Symptoms that may occur at this time are varied and may include any of the following:

- Mood swings and tearfulness for no apparent reason.

- Low energy levels and libido.

- Sleep disturbance or depression on waking.

- Lack of motivation.

- Panic attacks and palpitations.

- Lack of concentration.

- Poor appetite or overeating from boredom or needing comfort.

- Muscular tension and aches and pains.

Basic self-help measures

- Find ways of stimulating your interest in things and people outside the home. This can be a time when new opportunities present themselves in the form of adult education courses, learning new practical skills, enhancing and updating your current qualifications, or taking the opportunity to develop friendships that have dwindled. By exploring possibilities such as these, a situation that seems initially fruitless can be transformed into something exciting and give you a new lease of life.

- Focus on the positive benefits that maturity brings with it: greater experience, a more balanced perspective on life events, deeper emotional understanding and increased confidence. As many of us experience the

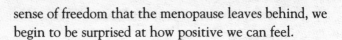

sense of freedom that the menopause leaves behind, we begin to be surprised at how positive we can feel.

• Be as honest as possible with your partner about how you feel. There is a strong possibility that you will be surprised at the impact it is also making on him. Men and women go through similar life crises at similar stages, but in the past, men have been conditioned not to show feelings of sadness, vulnerability, or despair. As a result, they have tended to cope by maintaining a stiff upper lip, or adopting a protective or emotionally superior role towards women, often at the cost of their own emotional release. This traditional male stance has been at the root of many tensions and misunderstandings between the sexes, often leading to a total breakdown in communication. Thankfully, things have slowly begun to change, with increasingly large numbers of men refusing to conform to stereotyped notions of masculinity, with their attendant problems of emotional suppression. By being honest, frank and open with your partner about your fears, insecurities and confusion regarding the ageing process, you may be surprised to find how positive the outcome might be with regard to a shared understanding of the situation.

• If symptoms are causing marked distress or do not improve as time goes by, you may gain great benefit from counselling. The latter is often of immense help in providing a wider perspective on how you feel.

• Make sure you are not neglecting your diet and that you are gaining maximum benefit from nutritious foods. Avoid food and drinks that are likely to make mood swings worse: these include alcohol, coffee, very sugary

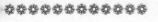

items like chocolate and biscuits, and fast foods. If you suspect you need a temporary boost, you may consider a good multi vitamin supplement, or a short course of high potency vitamin B-complex or vitamin C.

• Become more physically active. It has been demonstrated that regular, rhythmic exercise stimulates chemicals in our bodies that fulfil the role of natural antidepressants. It is the secretion of these chemicals that is understood to be responsible for the 'high' we experience after vigorous aerobic activity where our bodies make maximum use of the oxygen we breathe in. Not only does this make us feel good from a biochemical perspective, but it also makes us feel very positive about our bodies and general physical performance. The latter are both powerful confidence boosters at a time when our self-esteem can be at a rather low ebb.

Conventional treatment

If symptoms are severe and causing general disruption, the possible options include counselling or psychotherapy, tranquillisers or antidepressants.

Homoeopathic treatment

If your symptoms are mild and infrequent in nature, the self-help measures outlined above, plus an occasional dose of an appropriately selected homoeopathic medicine from the table below, may be all that is necessary to help you through a difficult time. However, if you feel that your symptoms are preventing you from getting on with your day-to-day life, if they seem to be getting worse, or if you find you need to repeat your homoeopathic medicine frequently to gain, or

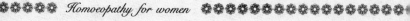

sustain improvement, you need to seek help from a trained practitioner. This also applies to anyone who has suffered from long-term anxiety or depression in the past. The latter would constitute a chronic emotional condition which should not be treated by self-prescribing. Because homoeopaths treat the whole person, mental, emotional and physical symptoms are all taken into consideration. As a result, disturbances involving emotional well-being pose no particular difficulty with regard to treatment.

TYPE	GENERAL INDICATIONS	WORSE FROM	BETTER FOR	REMEDY NAME
Anxiety with panic that comes and goes abruptly	Sudden feelings of fear that descend for no apparent reason. Terror, or conviction that death is near. Very restless, especially at night: fearful of the dark. Feels much worse for extreme heat or cold. Afraid of crowds and of going out.	At night. Extreme heat or cold. Becoming chilled. Stimulants	Fresh air. After sound sleep	Aconite
Anxiety and restlessness with fear of loss of control	Sense of unease and threat from disorder or untidiness. Fixated about own state of health, or health of family. Apprehensive and distressed by change: needs to feel in control by sticking to routine. When distressed, reacts very badly to being cold, comforted by warmth.	At night. Cold in any form. Being alone	Warmth. Sips of warm drinks. Movement	Arsenicum album

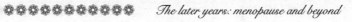

TYPE	GENERAL INDICATIONS	WORSE FROM	BETTER FOR	REMEDY NAME
Feeling low with irritability and no interest in family	Very physically and mentally exhausted. Lack of interest in partner with loss of libido, or positive aversion to making love. Fears being alone, but feels worse in company. Feels out of control and unable to cope.	Sitting still. Emotional demands. Humidity. Going without a meal	Vigorous exercise. Fresh, open air. Warmth. Sound sleep. Eating small amounts regularly	Sepia
Extreme feelings of stress and 'burn out' with irritability	Needed when commitment to work has become a substitute for home life. Works into the night and cannot switch off to get to sleep. May rely on stimulants to keep going, leading to anxiety and palpitations. Eats badly and drinks too much alcohol, resulting in constipation, indigestion and nausea.	In the morning. Being disturbed when asleep. Stimulants. Cold draughts. Alcohol, painkillers or sleeping pills. Touch. Mental or physical over-exertion	Sound sleep. Warmth. As the day goes on. Lying down	Nux vomica

TYPE	GENERAL INDICATIONS	WORSE FROM	BETTER FOR	REMEDY NAME
Sadness and depression from suppressed emotions	Withdrawn, antisocial and weepy in private. Reacts very badly to sympathy and attention: wants to be left alone. Mood swings may change rapidly from sadness to excitement. Feels worse for emotional release which feels demeaning, especially if it has occurred in front of others.	Sympathy. Warm, stuffy rooms. Touch or physical affection. Emotional stress. Physical effort. After sleep	Skipping meals. Being alone. Gentle exercise. Fresh, cool air	Natrum mur
'Free-floating anxiety' which attaches itself to anything	Emotionally sensitive and liable to pick up moods from others. Very responsive to attention and reassurance: very quickly made to feel calmer by a steadying influence. Inclined to get enthusiastic quickly, but bored or exhausted, equally rapidly.	Cold. Storms. Darkness. Evenings. Being alone. Crowds. Over-excitement	Reassur-ance. Warmth. Eating. Sound sleep. Massage	Phosphorus

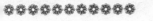

TYPE	GENERAL INDICATIONS	WORSE FROM	BETTER FOR	REMEDY NAME
Depressed and apathetic from suppressed anger towards family	Keeps a stiff upper lip: outwardly caring, considerate, reasonable and in control of emotions, while inwardly broods, fumes and dwells on resentments and injustices. Gets very angry over trivia, but avoids confronting roots of resentment and unhappiness. Feels violated after sexual contact.	Anger. Slight touch or pressure. Sexual activity. Smoking. Early morning	Eating. Warmth. Resting	Staphysagria
Moody and tearful with craving for sympathy and company	Weeps at slightest cause: feels much better for a good cry on a sympathetic shoulder. Moods are very variable and can be changed for the better by being in company. Fearful of the dark and being left alone. Insecure with need for reassurance.	Being alone. Darkness. At night. Stuffy, warm rooms. Humidity. Resting. Feeling neglected	Fresh, cool air. Gentle exercise out of doors. Cool bathing. Sympathy. A good cry. Physical affection. Uncovering	Pulsatilla

TYPE	GENERAL INDICATIONS	WORSE FROM	BETTER FOR	REMEDY NAME
Uncontrollable, and involuntary weepiness with strong mood swings	Very weepy and emotionally reactive after emotional stress or sense of bereavement. Erratic eating patterns when distressed with sleeping problems. Contradictory symptoms alternate between weepiness and excitement, being silent and talkative, or wanting company and demanding time alone.	Cold. Sugary foods. Cigarette smoke. Coffee. Emotional strain	Warmth. Eating. Activities that distract the mind from problems and distress	Ignatia

If symptoms are severe or long-standing, professional help is needed.

Heavy Bleeding

In the years approaching and during the menopause, we may experience a number of possible changes in our menstrual flow. One possible reaction is the abrupt cessation of periods, another is the setting in of a very irregular pattern, or we may find that our periods continue at ever-lengthening cycles, until we reach the point where they have stopped altogether. The nature of the flow may also change, with our periods either becoming very light and scanty, or very commonly heavy and gushing. The latter can be very frightening and debilitating, especially if we experience our

periods at regular intervals. Symptoms which may accompany flooding include:

• Very heavy bleeding that comes in gushes which seeps through regular sanitary protection. When severe, it may feel almost like a haemorrhage.

• Pains may also be very severe.

• Faintness and weakness.

• Nausea, vomiting, constipation or diarrhoea.

Basic self-help measures

• Take regular, moderate exercise that is also stress-relieving.

• Increase your intake of fresh, whole foods including large helpings of raw fruit and vegetables.

• Cut down on dairy foods, milk, alcohol, strong tea and coffee.

• If you suspect you may be anaemic (lacking in iron), make sure you include the following foods in your diet: eggs, fish, pulses, oatmeal, molasses, wholemeal bread, nuts, seeds, and green vegetables. Symptoms of anaemia include:

   • Exhaustion.
   • Pale complexion.
   • Palpitations.
   • Breathlessness.

Conventional treatment

Investigative tests may be suggested in order to establish whether the heavy bleeding is caused by fibroids. These ar benign lumps of muscle cells that cluster in the womb. Othe options to discount are endometriosis (see pages 85–87), or pelvic inflammatory disease (PID). If a D and C (Dilatation and Curettage) is suggested, this is an exploratory procedure that involves scraping the womb. If your GP suspects you are anaemic, you are also likely to be offered iron tablets. If despite all other efforts to relieve the problem bleeding continues to be very severe, you may be offered the option o a hysterectomy.

Homoeopathic treatment

As with other menstrual problems, homoeopathy has a vast amount to contribute in alleviating the distress an fear that are brought about by this condition. If bleeding is severe and protracted, it is necessary to seek professional advice in tackling the problem, rather than attempting to deal with it yourself. A homoeopath will place your menstrual symptoms within the broader context of your overall health and medical history in an effort to deal with underlying imbalances that may have contributed to the current problem. On the basis of this information, a prescription will be selected to fit your unique combination of symptoms with a view to enhancing the quality of your overall health and well-being, as well as improving your specific menstrual problems.

Professional advice should be sought if any of the followin occur:

- Severe or persistent symptoms.

- Bleeding or 'spotting' between periods.

- Any sign of bleeding after your periods have stopped.

Joint Pains and Arthritis

Women can suffer from a variety of muscle and joint-related problems during the course of their lives. These can vary from vague aches and pains and lack of flexibility to full-blown arthritis. Specific bone-related problems such as osteoporosis (brittle bones) can also become a problem in the years that follow the menopause, especially if we experience menopausal symptoms at an early age.

However, there is a positive side to this rather bleak picture since there are definite steps we can take at an early age to keep ourselves flexible and mobile well into our middle years and beyond. The foods we eat and the amount of exercise we take have an enormous impact on the health and resilience of our bones and joints. Conversely, a sedentary life and a high daily intake of foods that are known to aggravate joint problems, such as a high intake of refined foods, red meat and citrus fruits, is likely to encourage problems to develop.

The symptoms of osteoarthritis can arise any time around our forties and include:

- Restricted mobility as a result of pain and stiffness on movement.

- In severe or advanced cases the joint may look

misshapen due to degeneration of the cartilage and thickening of bone.

• Joints most likely to be affected are the large weight-bearing ones: these include the hips, knees and spine.

The symptoms of rheumatoid arthritis can arise at any time from childhood onwards. These include:

• Redness and inflammation in and around the affected joints.

• Swelling around the painful area.

• A hot sensation in the joint, or the painful area feels hot to the touch.

• General feelings of unwellness, weakness, feverishness and fatigue.

• Joints most likely to be affected include the fingers, wrists, toes, neck, and knees.

Predisposing factors

• Being overweight puts extra strain on the weight-bearing joints such as the hips and knees and encourages osteoarthritic problems.

• A diet high in coffee, tea, alcohol, dairy products, red meat and refined foods that combine large quantities of fat and sugar, such as cakes, biscuits and puddings, may all contribute to joint problems.

• Chronic constipation and laxative abuse may also play their part.

• A lifestyle that is overloaded with stress may also

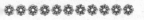

contribute to joint problems, especially if this results in relying on junk foods and stimulants to keep going, and alcohol to unwind. An overly demanding lifestyle can also result in little spare time being available for relaxation and exercise.

• Lack of exercise can also lead to overall stiffness, lack of muscle tone and flexibility.

Basic self-help measures

• Cut out or reduce greatly the amount of animal fat in your diet. Consider the feasibility of adopting a vegetarian eating plan for a trial period. Eat large helpings of salads with fresh, grated, raw vegetables, but avoid the following which belong to the nightshade family: green peppers, aubergine, tomatoes, and potatoes. Other foods which are believed to aggravate joint problems include dairy products, sugar, citrus fruits and wheat.

• Concentrate on light, low fat sources of protein such as fish or occasional portions of chicken (always choose white meat, i.e. breast, and avoid eating the skin) if becoming vegetarian is not a realistic option for you. However, make sure you greatly increase the fresh fruit and vegetable content of your diet by having a large helping of salad with each main meal. Substitute fresh fruit for puddings which are high in fat and sugar.

• Consider taking a vitamin C, B-complex and a fish oil supplement. Some sources suggest that extracts of the green-lipped mussel may also be helpful in relieving pain and inflammation.

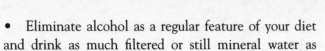

• Eliminate alcohol as a regular feature of your diet and drink as much filtered or still mineral water as possible in order to flush toxic waste out of your system: aim for six or eight large glasses daily.

• Massage can be a valuable aid to relaxation and pain relief, especially when used in conjunction with essential oils. However, be aware that some oils may interfere with the action of homoeopathic medicines. These include peppermint, camphor, eucalyptus, rosemary and thyme.

• Incorporate some form of exercise on a daily basis, especially if you have a sedentary job. Easy ways of introducing more exercise include opting for stairs rather than lifts, walking rather than using a car or public transport when going short distances, and taking walks as a way of unwinding and relaxing. If you are suffering from moderate stiffness in your joints it is essential to choose the most appropriate form of activity so that you don't unwittingly aggravate the condition. Swimming is often a beneficial exercise because the joints are supported in the water as you move, causing less pain and discomfort. However, be careful that you do not overdo it, and take things slowly. Avoid any form of activity that puts further strain on your joints through repetitive jarring motion: this would include jogging or running. Consider activities that encourage building strength, stamina and flexibility such as yoga, avoiding any postures that may put undue strain on your joints such as The Cat or The Triangle.

• Use Dead Sea Salt, Mud or Seaweed preparations

for a soothing and de-toxifying bath. Ensure that you use tepid water with powdered seaweed for maximum relaxing effect: if the water is too hot your heart rate may speed up uncomfortably, leading to palpitations.

Conventional treatment

Depending on the severity of the problem the possible medication may vary between painkillers, anti-inflammatories, or steroids. Other options may include physiotherapy or replacement of severely worn and damaged joints, such as the hip.

Homoeopathic treatment

The following table lists some of the most commonly indicated homoeopathic medicines for joint pain. If you suffer from occasional twinges, you will find the most appropriate remedy that fits your individual symptoms can give you effective and prompt relief from discomfort. However, if you need to take your remedy on a long-term basis to remain comfortable, or if you suspect that a more chronic problem is developing, it is essential to seek help from a homoeopathic practitioner in order to prevent further deterioration occurring. Through careful homoeopathic prescribing and other holistic measures it is often possible to minimise pain and prevent further destruction of bony tissue without the undesirable side-effects of conventional medication.

TYPE	GENERAL INDICATIONS	WORSE FROM	BETTER FOR	REMEDY NAME
Pale red, swollen joints that are much worse for any movement	Irritable, restless and bad-tempered with pains. General tendency to constipation, marked thirst and headaches. Generally responds well to cool things and badly to warm, but joints feel better for warmth. Joints are better on waking after rest and worse as the day goes on. Pains respond well to firm pressure.	Any effort. Standing or sitting. Getting up from sitting	Lying motionless. Firm pressure. Lying on the painful area	Bryonia
Pains that are better for continued movement	Very restless and depressed with discomfort. Painful joints that feel better for mild exercise, provided it doesn't go on too long and is not over-strenuous. Pains are worse on initial movement and better for being limbered up and warmth.	Cold. Damp. Resting. Lying or standing still. At night. Over-exertion	Warmth. Heat applied locally. Warm, dry weather. Continued movement	Rhus tox

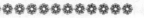 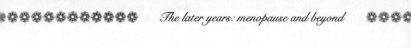

TYPE	GENERAL INDICATIONS	WORSE FROM	BETTER FOR	REMEDY NAME
Stiffness and pains that are much worse from heat	Weepy and in need of sympathy when in pain. Heavy sensations and aching in legs, especially at night. Changeable, wandering pains that migrate from joint to joint. Feels better for gentle movement in the open air.	Warmth. Stuffy rooms. Rest. At night. Heavy clothing or too heavy bedclothes. Getting chilled and wet	Fresh, open air. Gentle motion. Sympathy and attention. Lying on painful part. Cool in any form. Uncovering	Pulsatilla
Pains which are pricking and burning with very puffy swellings around joints	Very irritable and restless with pains. Swelling is rosy-red with a water-logged appearance which pits on pressure. All pains are much worse from exposure to heat and relieved by cold.	Warmth in any form. Hot bathing. Getting wet. Touch or pressure. Lying down. Keeping still. After sleep	Cool air. Cool bathing. Being uncovered. Walking	Apis
Joint pains that follow bites or stings or which are worse after a steroid injection	Joints look swollen and feel hot to the touch but do not look red. Stiffness and pain which is greatly relieved by cold bathing. Sore feet and heels after getting damp, made much worse by walking. Whole body aches and feels bruised.	Heat of bed. Too much clothing. Motion. Alcohol. After a warm bath. At night	Cool, open air. Bathing feet in very cold water. Cool applications. Resting	Ledum

TYPE	GENERAL INDICATIONS	WORSE FROM	BETTER FOR	REMEDY NAME
Joint pains with stinging, sharp sensations and hyper-sensitivity to pain	Great irritability and anger with pains: emotions are often bottled-up. Aching bones at night and a general sense of weariness in the limbs. Trembling and numbness of affected parts with bruised feelings.	Emotional strain. Touch. Pressure. Early morning	Eating. Resting. Warmth	Staphysagria

If joint pains are persistent and do not respond to self-help measures, or there is heat, swelling and inflammation of the joint, professional help should be sought.

CHAPTER 7

COMMON QUESTIONS ABOUT HOMOEOPATHIC TREATMENT

Is there any risk of homoeopathic medicines producing side-effects?

Because homoeopathic medicines are understood to work by stimulating the self-healing potential of the body by boosting vital energy, side-effects resulting from a toxic build-up are unlikely to happen. However, it is wise to be aware that over-stimulation from too enthusiastic a repetition of a homoeopathic medicine is always something to be avoided. It is for this reason that you should always stop and wait after giving a remedy if you have observed any reaction. Even slight improvement in symptoms is a sign that the body has been stimulated in the direction of a curative response, and that it can cope well under its own steam unless, or until, a relapse occurs. If the latter should happen, you can repeat the remedy again until you see evidence of further improvement. Once this happens, always watch and wait rather than repeating the remedy.

If a remedy has initially been very helpful but seems to have stopped being useful, take a closer look at the current symptoms and see if another remedy is now better indicated. If the symptoms have not changed, consider using a higher

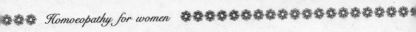

(stronger) potency of the original remedy.

The main problem with too frequent repetition of a homoeopathic medicine is that the original symptoms for which the remedy was given might get briefly more intense. If this happens, all that needs to be done is to withhold the remedy, and within a short space of time, things should return to where they were before the aggravation set in. On the other hand, if you continue to repeat an inappropriately chosen remedy for a relatively short period of time (for instance, two or three doses over the same number of hours) the worst that is likely to happen is the disappointment of seeing no improvement in the symptoms. In this situation there is no need to panic since no harm has been done. Just return to the remedy table and take a closer look at the symptoms to see if another remedy matches the symptoms more closely.

What if I am already taking orthodox medication such as antibiotics?

Competently prescribed homoeopathic medicines can be immensely useful in aiding the body in fighting bacterial or viral infections. The results obtained will depend very much on the skill and experience of the prescriber, but appropriate use of homoeopathic medicines as a first resort often means that antibiotics can be reserved for major infections that refuse to yield to more holistic, gentler measures.

Although it is much more straightforward and desirable to prescribe homoeopathically for someone who is not taking any conventional drugs, the practicalities of life often dictate otherwise. While it is far from ideal, it is still worth prescribing homoeopathically at home, especially if there are clear indications for an obvious remedy.

Although antibiotics and other drugs may interfere with the effective action of homoeopathic medicines, you don't need to worry about conventional medication and homoeopathic medicines having an adverse toxic interaction. This is because homoeopathic medication works on the energy levels of the patient, leaving no detectable chemical traces in the organs or bloodstream.

You can consider making an appointment with a homoeopath after the course of drugs is completed, especially if you feel that repeated courses of conventional medication are being prescribed on a frequent basis for recurrent infections. If homoeopathic treatment is successful, you should discover that illnesses are thrown off more decisively, resulting in fewer and less severe bouts of infection.

If you are considering home prescribing or general self-help measures and are on a course of conventional treatment which involves the use of steroids, never stop these drugs abruptly. There are many conventional drugs which require careful monitoring if they are to be reduced, and this should only be done with the full knowledge and co-operation of your GP.

How do I find a homoeopathic practitioner?

You can obtain registers of qualified homoeopathic practitioners from the following sources. The Society of Homoeopaths will supply you with a register of professional homoeopaths who have undergone a minimum of four years' training at an approved college. These practitioners are entitled to use the initials RS Hom.

If you require a list of orthodox doctors who also practise homoeopathy, you should contact the British Homoeopathic

Association. These practitioners are entitled to use the initials MF Hom.

Although registers are very useful in providing a basic guide to the qualifications held by individual practitioners in your area, the best method of locating a reputable homoeopath tends to be 'word of mouth'. In other words, if a friend, family member, or colleague at work has obtained homoeopathic treatment from a practitioner they found professional, knowledgeable, approachable, sympathetic and sensitive to their needs, it would be worth following this up with an enquiry. Bear in mind that the relationship that develops between practitioner and patient will always be unique, and what works for one person may not work for another. However, a strong personal recommendation can be of immense value in pointing you in the right direction as you begin enquiries.

This method is also an excellent way of taking into account that there are homoeopathic practitioners who trained before the college system was set up, who as a result may not always be included on available registers.

You can also consider looking through your local Yellow Pages entry under Homoeopathic Practitioners. This is not as ideal as as a strong personal recommendation for the reasons given above, but if it is all that is available to you, look for the initials mentioned in the first two paragraphs.

If you feel you have specific concerns about treatment, you can consider making a telephone enquiry. This will provide you with an opportunity to discuss briefly the relevant issues with the practitioner's receptionist, or in some cases, with the practitioner in person. This is also a useful way of finding about practical information, such as how long the initial consultation and follow-up appointments will be, and can also provide you with information about the basic costs involved.

What should I expect on my first visit to a homoeopath?

Many people find the initial consultation with a homoeopath is surprisingly lengthy since it normally takes between one to one and a half hours. This interview will be very thorough, with the homoeopath requiring detailed information about the current problem, general quality of health, current medication, medical history, and as accurate a picture as possible of emotional and psychological well-being within the limits of the time available. If your practitioner is also an orthodox doctor he or she might also want to conduct any appropriate physical examinations or tests.

After taking as full and detailed a case history as possible, your homoeopath will analyse the information as a whole, identifying the unifying features that run through your symptoms. On the basis of this analysis, your practitioner will select an appropriate homoeopathic medicine that matches your symptoms most closely on mental, emotional, and physical levels. The remedy may be given as a single tablet, or a short course of tablets that may be taken daily. Other methods of administration include powders, liquids or pilules. Once you have established your reaction to treatment, and communicated this to your practitioner, a decision will be made whether to wait, repeat the remedy, or change the prescription. You are likely to need to return for follow-up appointments every four to six weeks for the first few months in order to give your homoeopath a chance to assess your progress.

Are there situations where homoeopathy might not be of use?

Generally speaking, homoeopathic prescribing is of value in any of the conditions discussed in this book. Categories of problems where homoeopathic treatment would be likely to produce disappointing results might include any situation where permanent tissue damage has occurred, problems involving a mechanical obstacle to recovery, such as displaced vertebrae, or situations where so much strong orthodox medication has been taken that it is difficult to establish which are the patient's original symptoms and which are the result of side-effects of drug therapy.

However, even in some of the situations mentioned above, it is worth bearing in mind that homoeopathic prescribing may still be of value in minimising pain and distress as a useful adjunct to other therapies.

Can I combine homoeopathic treatment with other alternative therapies?

The majority of therapies that fall into the 'alternative' category such as massage, osteopathy, chiropractic, reflexology, or autogenic training, can be used side-by-side with homoeopathy. Any therapy which has at its heart the aim of helping the individual to achieve and maintain the maximum amount of balance and harmony between body and mind has a very similar aim to homoeopathy as a healing system. Yoga and the Alexander Technique may also both be helpful in teaching the homoeopathic patient more about the way they move and respond to stress, while basic relaxation techniques have a positive role to play in helping

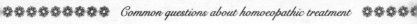

someone come to terms with the amount of mental and emotional strain they have in their lives.

It has been suggested that acupuncture, although it has much in common with homoeopathy as a holistic system of medicine, may not work compatibly with homoeopathic treatment. In these cases, it is often suggested that the patient concentrates on one of these two therapies for a while in order to assess the benefits of each independently.

Once you begin to experience homoeopathy as a system of healing for yourself and others, it is noticeable that a natural examination of diet and lifestyle begins. This is a very positive development, since there is little point in substituting homoeopathic medicines for orthodox drugs if there is an underlying factor that is leading to the problem, such as too high a consumption of alcohol, or a highly indigestible or poorly nourished diet. This does not mean that you have to become a strict vegetarian overnight, or give up alcohol or other foods that give pleasure in moderation: a harsh or guilt-ridden approach will not lead to a sense of balance either. However, as you become more familiar with the factors that lead your body to experience a sense of enhanced well-being, and those that do the reverse, the chances are that you will want to take the chance to maximise your optimum level of health and vitality by supporting your body, rather than fighting against it.

KEYNOTES

Please refer to the relevant section in the chapter
Homoeopathy in Action on how to use this section.

Aconite

Often needed in the early stages (the first twenty-four to
forty-eight hours) of a quickly developing problem.
Especially indicated where there is anxiety, fever and
restlessness. Problems often follow becoming chilled,
exposure to dry, cold winds, or severe emotional trauma.
Also very appropriate for the fear and 'nerves' that often
precede admission to hospital for surgery: especially where
there is a strong conviction that something is bound to go
wrong.

Mental/Emotional Picture
- Awfully anxious and fearful to the point of terror and
  panic: convinced that she is about to die.
- Symptoms often follow rapidly after emotional shock or
  trauma.
- Terrific sensitivity on mental, emotional and physical
  levels.
- Pains are intolerable, with strong aversion to being
  approached or touched.
- Frequent panic attacks with specific fear of crowds, open
  spaces, and the dark.

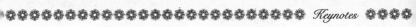

Fever

- Very sudden onset of high temperature and flushes of heat with hot head and cold body.
- Fever and inflammation follows on violently and rapidly after being exposed to dry, cold winds, or becoming chilled.
- Symptoms may subside as rapidly as they set in.

Head

- Headaches develop suddenly with high temperature and shivering.
- Giddiness or headache may be brought on by an upsetting or frightening experience.

Eyes

- Symptoms develop very rapidly and violently.
- Over-sensitivity to light with burning, watering and redness.
- Often useful in eye injuries where there is swelling and burning.

Nose and Throat

- Nose runs after exposure to chill or cold winds.
- Nasal discharge is clear, fluent, and hot.
- Nasal passages are much more comfortable for being out of doors in the fresh air.
- Difficulty swallowing with dry, hoarse, tingling throat.
- Tight, constricted sensation in throat when swallowing.

Chest

- Dry, barking cough that is brought on by exposure to cold winds.
- Wakes frequently at night with violent cough and choking fits.

- Cough is worse from being upset, during the night, talking, eating or drinking.

Digestion
- Sudden onset of upset stomach after emotional trauma.
- Sudden appearance of diarrhoea after shock.
- Very restless with marked tenderness around region of stomach that is aggravated by moving.
- Marked thirst for water, which is the only thing that does not taste bitter.

Kidneys and Bladder
- Sudden onset of violent, cutting, tearing pains.
- Concentrated, dark, and possibly bloody urine which feels hot to pass.
- Urination problems in newborn babies.

Reproductive Organs
- Menstrual problems may date back from a time of stress, fear or shock.
- Severe pains which feel cutting, stabbing or tearing.
- 'Beside herself' with the pains which feel unbearable.
- Flushes of heat, numbness or tingling with pains.
- Flow is gushing and bright in colour.
- Panic with heavy bleeding.

Sleep
- Drowsy during the day but sleepless at night.
- Tosses and turns with restless sleep.
- Disturbed sleep pattern often follows being involved in, or witnessing, an accident.
- Fitful sleep with terrors and nightmares.

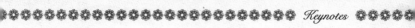

Skin

• Extra-sensitive skin with slightest touch causing discomfort.

Worse from	*Better for*
Extreme hot or cold	Undisturbed sleep
Exposure to chill or dry, cold winds	Fresh air
Fright or shock	Sweating
At night	
Warm, stuffy rooms	
Lying on painful part	

Apis

Particularly indicated in situations of extreme allergic reactions involving rapid swelling, inflammation and accumulation of fluid in the tissues.

Mental/Emotional Picture

• Problems may set in after a period of stress or emotional upset.
• Hypersensitive to least touch or physical contact.
• Very fidgety, irritable and fussy.

Fever

• Very much worse for contact with heat in any form and much more comfortable for cool applications and fresh air.
• Although temperature may be high, there is a marked absence of thirst.
• Chilled and thirsty once fever subsides.

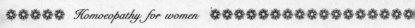

Head
- Headaches much worse for jarring and warm surroundings.
- Hot head and throbbing pains with headache.

Eyes
- Violent and sudden puffy swelling of eyelids: 'water bag' swelling beneath the eyes,
- Light sensitivity with watering eyes.
- Cool bathing eases discomfort and swelling temporarily.

Nose and Throat
- Allergic reactions with violent sneezing.
- Nostrils may be permanently blocked, or there might be scanty nasal discharge.
- Throat swells and uvula looks puffy and swollen.
- Inflammation makes the throat look water-logged or 'glossy' in appearance.
- Difficulty in swallowing: even sips of water are difficult to swallow.
- Tight, constricted sensation in throat.

Chest
- Suffocative sensations in a warm, stuffy room.
- Breathing difficulties are made worse by leaning forwards or backwards.

Digestion
- Tense, swollen stomach that is very sensitive to touch or slight contact.
- Sneezing aggravates burning pains in stomach.
- Raw, burning sensations after diarrhoea which are relieved and soothed by cool bathing.

Kidneys and Bladder
- Scanty, concentrated urine that burns as it is being passed.
- Fluid retention associated with urinary disorders, especially around the eyes which look very puffy.
- General sense of aching, soreness, and discomfort with bladder and kidney problems.
- Lack of thirst with urinary disorders.

Reproductive Organs
- Ovarian pain with marked discomfort on the right side which may spread to the left.
- Pains are characteristically burning and stinging.

Sleep
- Cannot get comfortable in bed if overheated.
- Tosses and turns and throws covers off in an effort to cool down.
- May cry out in restless sleep.

Skin
- Pink, puffy, raised blotches that look as though water is trapped beneath the skin.
- Stinging and itching sensations are much relieved by cool bathing and contact with cool air, and made much worse by exposure to heat in any form.
- Often needed in cases of hives that come on after being overheated.

Worse from	*Better for*
Heat in any form including hot bathing, fires, or overwarm rooms	Cold in any form: air, applications, bathing, or uncovering
Touch or contact	Moving about in the fresh, cool air
Warm drinks	

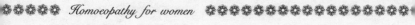
Resting	Sitting up
Lying down	
After sleep	
At night	

Arnica

The first remedy to administer in any cases of bruising, shock, accident, or trauma of any kind. It helps stop bleeding, encourages healing and the re-absorption of blood from bruised tissues. Consider it before and after dental work, muscle strains, early stages of a fracture, after childbirth, or for generalised aching after muscular overexertion.

Mental/Emotional Picture
- Pushes people away during the immediate shock following an accident or fall: insists she just wants to be left alone.
- Aching pains and extreme physical sensitivity: dislikes anyone approaching because of aversion to being touched.
- Irritable, restless, and short-tempered with pain.

Head
- Nauseated with one-sided headache.
- Giddiness on waking or moving which is worse when eyes are closed.

Eyes
- Burning sensations with conjunctivitis or eye strain.
- Bleeding or bruising after injury.

Nose and Throat
- Nosebleeds follow injury with tingling in nose.
- Bruised or aching sensations in throat.

Chest
- Dry, tickly cough that is worse in the mornings.
- Stitching pains in the chest that are aggravated by moving and coughing.

Digestion
- Excessive amounts of saliva with nausea.
- Involuntary passage of diarrhoea.
- Abdominal, colicky pains in the abdomen with accompanying wind.

Kidneys and Bladder
- Urine may be retained after overexertion.
- Difficult passage of urine although there is a frequent urge to do so.
- May have to wait for a while before flow of urine begins.

Reproductive Organs
- Severe pains which may be especially severe at night.
- General state of exhaustion during the menopause with flushes of heat to head, cold body, and palpitations.

Sleep
- Aches all over with tiredness.
- Very restless: bed feels much too hard to rest in.
- Difficulty getting to sleep until the early hours of the morning: once asleep, wakes frequently from bad dreams.

Skin
- Aching soreness and bruising with tenderness.
- General aching, throbbing and burning pains with exhaustion after overexertion.
- Indicated for boils or abscesses that are very painful but refuse to come to a head.

Worse from	Better for
Movement	Lying undisturbed with head
Being approached	lower than body
Touch	
Damp	
Cold	

Arsenicum album

Mental/Emotional Picture

- Very anxious, restless and exhausted with illness.
- Even though feeling mentally, emotionally and physically exhausted, cannot rest if surroundings are untidy or in need of cleaning.
- Over-sensitive and fussy about everything.
- Terribly physically and mentally restless.
- All symptoms are much worse for being alone, especially at night.
- Awful anxiety building up to a state of panic that gets steadily worse as the night goes on.
- Specific fears of the dark, death and serious illness.

Fever

- Very cold with feverishness: ice-cold sensations surge through the body.
- With high temperature feels as though she is burning up from head to foot, but generally feels better for warmth or heat applied locally.
- Feverish with desire for sips of warm drinks rather than large gulps of cool liquids.

Head

- Nausea and vomiting with headache.

- Headaches may develop in the afternoon and get steadily worse as the night goes on.
- The head is the only part of the body that is relieved by exposure to cool, fresh air; everything else is better for contact with warmth.

Eyes
- Terrible sensitivity to light with burning and redness of the eyes.
- Swelling of upper and lower lids.
- Discomfort in eyes is relieved by warmth.

Nose and Throat
- Scanty, burning, clear nasal discharge with violent sneezing.
- Acrid nasal discharge leaves the nostrils and upper lip red, burning and sore.
- Burning pains in the throat are soothed by sips of warm drinks.

Chest
- Asthmatic symptoms may develop as a result of panic, anxiety or stress.
- Wheezy and anxious with troublesome, dry, unproductive cough.
- Persistent cough is worse at night and better for sitting propped-up in bed in a warm atmosphere.
- Coughing spasms are aggravated by lying flat or being chilled out of doors.

Digestion
- Vomiting and diarrhoea occur together resulting in restless exhaustion and collapse.
- Indigestion and burning pains in stomach are relieved by warm drinks and warm applications.

- Sips of warm drinks are soothing while long cold drinks are vomited back immediately.
- Cannot bear the thought, sight, or smell of food.

Kidneys and Bladder
- Kidney problems may follow on from dehydration as a result of vomiting and diarrhoea occurring together.
- Burning sensations on passing urine.
- Generally chilly and/or feverish with kidney or bladder involvement.

Reproductive Organs
- Severe pain with diarrhoea and vomiting.
- Prostrated with pains but also constantly restless.
- Very chilly and pale.
- Pains are relieved by warmth in general, but also from heat applied locally to the painful area.

Sleep
- Drowsy by day and sleepless at night.
- Very mentally and physically restless at night when all symptoms are worse.
- May find it impossible to stay in bed and feels compelled to wander about.
- Wakes worrying about the things that have to be organised for the day ahead.

Skin
- Burning, itchy skin that feels much worse after scratching.
- Intense, compulsive scratching that causes weeping and bleeding of the skin.
- Rubbing makes the itching temporarily better, but burning is not improved.
- Eruptions on the skin feel better for contact with warmth.

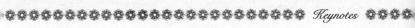

Worse from	*Better for*
Cold air, rooms, drinks and applications	Warm air, rooms, drinks and applications
Being alone	Company and distraction
At night: especially after midnight	Limited movement
Draughts	Company
Lying flat in bed	Fresh air improves headache

Belladonna

L ike *Aconite* this remedy is most often needed in the early stage of illness, inflammation or fever, especially when the symptoms have developed violently and rapidly. For the later, more established stage of illness, another remedy is likely to be needed.

Mental/Emotional Picture
- Irritable and short-tempered with onset of illness.
- Someone who is normally placid and easy-going becomes very aggressive and difficult to please if they are entering a Belladonna state.
- Alternation between over-excitability and drowsiness or lethargy.
- Adversely affected by stimulation of any kind such as noise, bright light, and jarring movement.
- May hallucinate with high temperature.
- More irritable and aggressive than anxious, fearful or panicky.

Fever
- Rapid, violent onset of high temperature with very hot, bright red, dry skin.

187

- Although very hot, feels worse for exposure to cold or being uncovered.
- Hot head and cold extremities.
- Covered parts of the body perspire.
- Very rapid, bounding pulse with high temperature.

Head

- Very sensitive scalp with violent, throbbing headaches: as a result, avoids having hair touched.
- Feels more comfortable bending head backwards.
- Unlike more general features of the remedy, headaches may feel better from cool applications and exposure to open, fresh air.
- Headache is worse lying flat, bending forwards, bright lights and jarring movements.

Eyes

- Dilated pupils and glassy eyes with high temperature.
- Eyes feel hot and look inflamed and red.
- Spasmodic, twitching movements of eyelids.

Nose and Throat

- Red, flushed face with red, swollen tip to nose.
- Extremely acute sense of smell with unpleasant odour in nasal passages.
- Very painful, dry, throbbing throat that makes the swallowing of liquids extremely difficult.
- Tonsils very inflamed, especially on the right side.
- Rapid hoarseness with complete loss of voice.

Chest

- Dry, barking cough that is much worse lying flat at night.
- Cough is temporarily relieved by bringing up mucus.
- Irritation and tickling in throat precedes coughing fit.

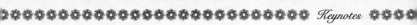

Digestion

- Cramping, colicky pains in digestive tract are relieved by bending forwards or backwards.
- Stomach and abdomen are hypersensitive to touch: even bed clothes and clothing cause distress and discomfort.
- Diarrhoea with constant urging.

Kidneys and Bladder

- Constant urge to urinate with distress from cutting and burning sensations.
- Retention of urine or constant dribbling and loss of bladder control.
- Constricting sensations and spasms felt in bladder after passing urine.
- Urine may be dark, bloody or cloudy.

Reproductive Organs

- Heavy bleeding with strong, painful contractions.
- Copious, hot, clotted flow which is bright in colour.
- Bearing-down sensations with, or without, actual prolapse.
- Right-sided ovarian pain.
- Periods may be early with extremely heavy flow.

Skin

- Very painful and hypersensitive skin.
- Dry, bright red skin so intensely flushed that it radiates heat.
- One of the major remedies to consider in cases of sunburn.

Worse from	*Better for*
Sensory stimulation of any kind	Resting undisturbed
Lying on painful, inflamed areas	Lying propped-up in a darkened room
	Warm, quiet surroundings

Cold   Bending head backwards
Draughts of cold air

Bryonia

Frequently indicated for situations that develop in a slow, insidious way: e.g. colds that get worse after a few days of feeling off-colour, or joint pains that get slowly worse.

Mental/Emotional Picture
- Very irritable, short-tempered and cross when disturbed.
- Discontented and difficult to please: asks for something and then rejects it.
- Wants to lie as still as possible in a quiet, cool room.
- Marked aversion to making any kind of physical effort.
- Angry at being unwell: just wants to get back to normal.
- Anxiety about finances, work, and general lack of security.

Fever
- Sweaty with fever during the night.
- Marked aversion to being wrapped-up warmly or to being in a warm room.
- Marked thirst when feverish for large quantities of cold water.

Head
- Headache may follow constipation.
- Severe frontal headache which is made worse by the slightest movement, and stooping.
- Instinctively holds on to the head to keep it as still as possible when in pain.
- Head pain is worse from heat and better for cool in any form.

Eyes

- Red, sore, inflamed eyes that feel worse for the slightest movement.
- Eyes feel hot and gritty.

Nose and Throat

- Pains in forehead with nasal discharge.
- Red, sore swelling of nose.
- General dryness of nasal passages with irritation extending to the throat and upper chest.
- Scanty mucus which is very difficult to raise.

Chest

- Coughing spasms are brought on by energising a warm atmosphere.
- Dry, tickling, irritating cough with possible gagging.
- Feels she wants to take a deep breath but this makes the cough worse.
- Pain is chest is relieved by firm pressure, so hand is pressed instinctively to the painful area in the chest or head when coughing.

Digestion

- Very parched mouth with marked thirst for cool drinks.
- Nausea is aggravated by eating and movement, and temporarily relieved by bringing up wind.
- Exhausting diarrhoea that is made much worse by the slightest movement.
- Diarrhoea may be brought on by eating too much acid fruit.
- Constipation with dry, large, hard stools that are very difficult to pass.

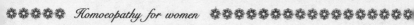

Bladder and Kidneys
- Dark-coloured urine that feels hot when it is being passed.
- Urgent desire to pass water with cutting pains.

Reproductive Organs
- Pain in groin before period begins.
- Burning pains when the flow starts.
- Periods may be delayed from stress or overexertion before the period is due.
- Very painful, enlarged breasts as part of a general picture of pre-menstrual syndrome.
- Mastitis with heavy, hot, painful breasts.

Sleep
- Very drowsy during the day with great difficulty sleeping at night.
- Unrefreshing sleep with a tendency to wake in a state of anxiety when dropping off to sleep.

Worse from	*Better for*
Warmth	Cool
Physical or mental effort	Lying as still as possible
Sitting up from lying down	Firm pressure to painful part
The slightest movement	Perspiring
Initial movement after resting	Resting

Calc carb

It is worth noting that this remedy is seldom indicated for short-lived, acute problems, and is most often used for long-term, far-reaching, constitutional treatment. Therefore it must be stressed that it is a remedy that does not require frequent repetition.

Mental/Emotional Picture
- Strong-willed, obstinate personalities who approach tasks with dogged determination at their own slow pace.
- Marked dislike of being rushed or hurried.
- Very poor long-term physical stamina: complete exhaustion sets in rapidly.
- Sensitive natures which are full of fears and insecurities including lack of confidence, fear of being alone, and anxiety in the dark.
- Very self-conscious with fear of other people seeing her confusion, insecurity or distress.
- Adverse reaction to criticism.
- Physical and mental reactions appear very slow: developmental milestones as an infant may have also been later than expected.

Fever
- Repeated pattern of constant infections in winter, such as colds, sore throats, ear infections, and swollen glands.
- Although easily overheated and flushed, hands and feet always feel icy, sweaty and excessively clammy.
- If feverish, sweats suddenly occur from exertion.
- Marked tendency to sweatiness, especially on scalp and feet when under bedclothes at night.

Head
- Nausea with headache that is relieved by warmth and made worse by cold or draughts of air.
- Discomfort generally eased by resting and taking it easy.

Eyes

- Easily strained eyes with resulting filmy or veiled sensation.
- Rapid tiredness of eye muscles from reading or watching television.

Nose and Throat

- Thick nasal discharge with sore nose.
- Recurrent and persistent winter sore throats with swollen glands.
- Painless hoarseness or loss of voice on waking.

Chest

- Irritating, tickly cough at night, or rattling, productive coughing spasms, with large amounts of thick, yellow mucus which has a sweet taste.

Digestion

- Sluggish digestion with stubborn constipation or alternation between diarrhoea and constipation.
- Unusual food cravings including chalk or coal. Others include pasta, eggs, bread, sweets and salt.
- Dislike of foods with a milky, slimy texture and hot dishes.
- Generally feels better when constipated.

Kidneys and Bladder

- Recurrent cystitis with concentrated, dark, brown-tinged urine that has a sour, unpleasant smell.

Reproductive Organs

- PMS with swollen, painful breasts before and during the period.
- Right-sided ovarian pain which extends to the thigh on the same side.

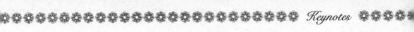

- Period may come early as a result of stress or overexertion.
- Pains are cramping and affect the stomach.
- Vaginal discharge is thick, itchy, burning, and sour-smelling.

Sleep
- Fitful, disturbed sleep with a tendency to recurrent bad dreams.
- Wakes so upset from sleep that it takes a long time to calm down.
- Sleepwalks or grinds teeth in sleep.

Skin
- Texture is generally dry and develops cracks or chaps during the winter months.
- Childhood history of chronic skin problems including eczema, nappy rash, urticaria, warts and cradle cap.

Worse from	*Better for*
Cold and wet	Warmth
Draughts of frosty air	Resting
Changes from warm to cold weather	Fine weather
	Moderate temperatures
Being observed	When constipated
Criticism	

Calendula

Mainly used as an external application in the form of lotion, cream, ointment, or diluted tincture. The antiseptic properties of this remedy make it an ideal skin

salve for wounds and abrasions since it promotes healing of
tissue, slows down bleeding, and helps prevent infection.

Cantharis

One of the main remedies to consider in cases of cystitis
where there are very few individualising symptoms.
Symptoms develop with violence and extreme rapidity.

Mental/Emotional Picture
- Thoughts may be confused to the point of seeming
  stupefied, or the mental state may be one of hyper-
  excitability or delirium.
- Marked irritability and bad-temper.
- Terrific hypersensitivity to any sensory stimulation
  including bright light or slight touch.

Fever
- Sensation of burning up or being on fire: this may develop
  into a state where internal burning is experienced, but
  the skin is cold to the touch.
- Cold sweat on extremities and genital organs.

Headache
- Violent, throbbing or stabbing pains with headache.
- Tension headaches which stem from the nape of the neck
  and feel better when walking about.

Eyes
- Burning sensations with conjunctivitis.

Nose and Throat
- Fluids are very difficult to swallow because of burning and
  rawness in throat.
- Constricted, tight feeling when drinking.

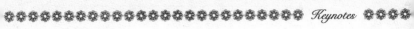

Chest
- Burning sensations in chest with copious, ropy mucus which is difficult to raise.

Digestion
- Violent burning in stomach with possible vomiting.
- May bend double in search of relief.
- Swollen, tender abdomen with watery diarrhoea.
- Feels the urge for a bowel movement when passing water.

Kidneys and Bladder
- Burning and cutting sensations before, during and after passing water.
- Similar sensations in the kidney region with accompanying tenderness.
- Acute distress on passing water with frequent urge to do so.

Reproductive Organs
- Burning ovarian pains.
- Increased sensitivity of genitals leads to increased libido and desire.

Sleep
- Although prostrated and drowsy by day, unable to sleep at night due to intense discomfort from symptoms.

Skin
- Especially indicated for internal use in burns and scalds, gnat bites or sunburn. Large blister formation with intense burning.

Worse from	*Better for*
Movement	Warmth
Touch	Passing wind
Drinking	At night
Coffee	

Carbo veg

Especially indicated for general symptoms of shock and collapse.

Mental/Emotional Picture
- Confused and withdrawn.
- Apathetic and indifferent to surroundings.
- Irritability.
- General anxiety with specific fear of the dark.

Fever
- Clammy, sweaty and chilly with craving for fresh air: asks to be fanned.
- Very pale with bluish tinge to the skin.
- Although cold to touch, may complain of feeling burning hot inside, especially inside the chest.

Head
- Throbbing pains in temples with headache.
- Sensation of a tight band around the head.
- Headaches feel worse from the least movement and effort.

Eyes
- Burning sensations in eyes with heavy feeling in lids.
- Edges of eyelids feel itchy.

Nose and Throat
- Frequent nosebleeds with sneezing.
- Reacts badly to extreme changes in temperature.
- General sensation of unwellness with mucus in nasal passages.
- Nose feels cold and sore and looks red at the tip.
- Hoarseness with burning sensations in throat.
- Throat pain is worse from talking, clearing the throat and exposure to damp air.

Chest

- Coughing spasms end in gagging or vomiting of mucus with flushing of the face.
- Suffocative sensations come on after lying down and are eased by contact with fresh air.
- Abundant, rattling mucus in the chest which is raised with great difficulty and effort.
- Feelings of burning and weakness in chest cause great distress.

Digestion

- Constant belching which only gives temporary relief.
- Burning sensations in the stomach.
- Nausea and general queasiness from overindulgence.
- Colicky pains with rumbling and diarrhoea.

Kidneys and Bladder

- Difficulty passing water after a night's rest.
- Constant, urgent, anxious desire to pass water day and night.
- Smarting sensations on passing water.
- Urine is scanty, deep-coloured, cloudy and reddish in appearance.

Reproductive Organs

- Early or very heavy periods with pale flow.
- Headaches and abdominal cramps before the period begins.
- Discharge before periods that is thick, white or yellowy-green.
- Itching, burning and general sensitivity with discharge.
- Exhaustion and milk slow to let down in breastfeeding mothers.

Sleep

- Twitches and jerks in light sleep.
- Wakes feeling clammy covered in perspiration.

Skin

- Burning sensations on the skin with a tendency to easy bruising.
- Rapid formation of ulcers.

Worse from	Better for
Warm, stuffy surroundings	Being fanned
Humidity	After sleep
Movement	Bringing wind up
After eating	Fresh, cool, open air
Cold	

Causticum

This remedy is of immense value to people who have gradually experienced a decline in their state of health. Problems especially affect the tendons and joints in the hands and feet leading to stiffness, deformities, and cramping pains. Sensations are characteristically raw, burning, sore and cramping.

Mental/Emotional Picture

- Timid, anxious and nervous.
- Hypersensitive to noise, touch or excitement.
- Intense sympathy with the sufferings of others: often motivated to defend others against unfair treatment or behaviour.
- Absent-minded with a poor memory.
- May become critical, suspicious or irritable.
- Often needed in cases of long-term emotional stress, grief, or worry which has slowly undermined the health.

Head

- Sick headache which is worse in a warm room.
- Tight, constricted feeling in scalp which is relieved by warmth.
- Dizziness with a tendency to fall to one side.
- Headaches with facial neuralgia or Bell's Palsy.

Eyes

- Gritty feeling with tendency to close the eyes.
- Heavy sensations in eyelids.

Nose and Throat

- Dry sensation in nostrils with stuffed-up sensation.
- Itching at tip of nose and in the nasal passages.
- Post-nasal drip which is thick and yellowy-green in colour.
- Raw, sore throat with hoarseness or complete loss of voice.
- Burning pains in throat are worse in the mornings.

Chest

- Irritating dry, hollow cough from tickling in the throat.
- Leakage of urine when coughing.
- Tight feelings in chest with cough with constant feeling of breathlessness.
- Coughing is eased by sips of cold water and aggravated by getting warm in bed.

Digestion

- Burning thirst for cold drinks.
- Acidity in stomach with nausea.
- Colicky pains are relieved by bending double and lying down.
- Haemorrhoids and anal fissure with itching or sticking pains.

- Involuntary passage of stool.

Kidneys and Bladder
- Stress incontinence is aggravated by coughing, sneezing or laughing.
- Frequent desire to pass large quantities of urine may lead to involuntary passage of urine when asleep.
- Cystitis with acute sensitivity to cold.

Reproductive Organs
- Delayed periods with heavy, clotted flow.
- Flow stops temporarily when lying down.
- Pale, dizzy and depressed before period.
- Lack of sexual interest from exhaustion.
- Vaginal discharge at night, but stops during the day.
- Scanty milk supply and cracked, sore nipples when breastfeeding.

Sleep
- Marked insomnia with restless legs.
- Sees frightening images on falling asleep and wakes with a start.
- Night is generally a very anxious time.
- Fear of the dark may have been present since childhood.

Skin
- Acne may affect the cheeks and forehead.
- Spots and eruptions behind the ears.
- Warts on the eyelids, face and hands which may bleed easily.
- Old scars remain sensitive and refuse to heal completely.
- Violent itching on the back and calves of the legs especially marked at night.

Worse from	*Better for*
Cold, dry winds	Warm, humid weather
The onset of cold weather	Getting warm in bed (except
Moving into a warm	for chest symptoms)
atmosphere	Cold drinks
Draughts	
After bathing	
Travelling in a car	
At night	
Drinking coffee	

Chamomilla

Mental/Emotional Picture
- Physically and emotionally over-sensitive.
- Aversion to being touched.
- Impatience and extreme frustration which leads to feelings of being out of control and violence.
- Throws things about in anger and frustration.
- Shouts and screams.
- Easily offended and refuses to reply to questions.
- Paces the floor to calm down.

Fever
- General flushed appearance: one cheek looks red and the other pale.
- Thirsty for cold drinks.
- Hot feet that are constantly moved about the bed in the search for a cold spot.
- Warm, moist head from perspiration.

Head
- Headache is caused by or made worse from feeling angry.

- Head generally feels better for being wrapped-up and from warmth in general.

Eyes
- Swollen eyes on waking with eyelids that stick together.

Nose and Throat
- Lots of dry, irritating sneezing.
- Obstructed, blocked nostrils with hot, watery discharge.

Chest
- Dry, hacking cough at night that is set off by talking.
- Disturbed sleep from coughing which leads to bad-temper on waking.
- Anger and frustration bring on a coughing fit.

Digestion
- Colicky pains that are not improved by passing wind, but which feel better from heat applied locally.
- Stomach pains result in instinct to draw knees up to chest when lying down.
- Watery, greenish-coloured diarrhoea with stomach pains.

Kidneys and Bladder
- Itching and burning when passing urine.
- Cloudy, yellowish, hot urine.

Reproductive Organs
- Severe irritability with PMS.
- Unbearable labour-like pains with period.
- Deep-red coloured flow which is clotted and heavy.
- Spotting between periods.
- Unbearable, insufficient labour pains that drive to distraction and fury.
- Very tender, enlarged breasts and sore, sensitive nipples.

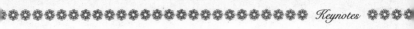

Sleep
- Disturbed, restless, poor quality sleep.
- Frequent bad dreams.
- Tosses, moans and starts in sleep.

Worse from	*Better for*
Exposure to wind and draughts	Warm, moist weather
Damp	Rocking movement
Before and during periods	Car travel
Anger and frustration	
Coffee and sedatives	

Cimicifuga

Mental/Emotional Picture
- Gloomy and depressed: feels as though a black cloud is looming over her.
- Terrible anxieties with specific fear of losing her reason.
- Very over-talkative: constantly chances topics.
- Fidgety and on-edge.
- Severe depression is much worse before a period.
- Sighs frequently.
- Often indicated after childbirth when black moods and depression may be very marked.

Head
- Awful migraines and headaches during the menopause.
- Frequent flushes of heat to the head.
- Severe pains at nape of neck which extend to the top of the head.
- Head pain is generally worse indoors and better in the open air.

Eyes

- Intense aching in the eyeballs that feels better for pressure and worse from the slightest movement.

Digestion

- Nausea with belching and headache.
- Sinking feelings in the stomach.
- Colicky pains that are better after a bowel movement and bending double.
- Alternation between diarrhoea and constipation.

Kidneys and Bladder

- Pressing pains in small of back and kidneys.
- Constant desire to pass water.

Reproductive Organs

- Very emotionally disturbed before and during periods.
- Feels strange and self-destructive.
- Pains shoot from side to side or upwards.
- Heavy, bearing-down sensations in womb and small of back.
- Nausea in pregnancy with false labour pains.
- Tendency to miscarry easily.
- Pains and inflammation in breasts: worse on the left side.
- Ineffective, shooting labour pains that seem to fly around all over the place.
- Sore, bruised pains in joints and in the lower back.
- Afterpains are severe with general hypersensitivity and intolerance of pain.

Sleep

- Very restless at night from rheumatic pains and specific pain in the neck.
- Sleeplessness with jerking limbs and restlessness.

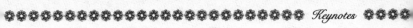

Worse from	*Better for*
Periods	Fresh air
Damp	Continued movement
Cold	Pressure
	Warmth

Gelsemium

Indicated for conditions that take a long time to develop, rather than those that emerge with violence and rapidity.

Mental/Emotional Picture

- Symptoms may be preceded by excitement, sudden fright, shock, or bad news.
- Mentally and physically weary, fatigued and exhausted.
- Cannot be bothered with anything: just wants to be left alone in peace.
- Unable to make the necessary effort to get involved in any activity that calls for effort or enthusiasm.
- Specific fear of the dark.

Fever

- Aversion to being in warm room even though feeling shivery with chills running up and down spine.
- When a sweat breaks out, it does nothing to relieve the general symptoms.
- Hot, flushed face and head with cold extremities.
- Muscular weakness and trembling with wobbly legs.

Head

- Specific sensation as though head was compressed by a tight band resting above the eyes.
- Sore scalp and shoulder muscles with headache.

- Pains in head feel worse for exposure to warmth and better for keeping still, ideally propped-up in bed.

Eyes
- Eyes feel heavy and lids look droopy and sagging during illness or tiredness.
- Blurred vision and dizziness with tiredness that are aggravated by motion.

Nose and Throat
- Slow, insidious development of cold or flu symptoms that begin with severe sneezing and hot nasal discharge.
- Complete obstruction of nasal passages with red, sore nostrils.
- Sore throat looks puffy, red and swollen.
- Pains shoot from the throat to the ear on swallowing.
- Sensation of lump in the throat which makes swallowing difficult and uncomfortable.

Chest
- Shallow breathing with sudden bouts of breathlessness.
- Sore chest from violent coughing spasms.

Digestion
- Painless diarrhoea as a result of anticipation or 'nerves'.
- Withdrawn and brooding with anxiety rather than chatty and talkative.
- Unusual feature of dry lips and mouth with no thirst.

Kidneys and Bladder
- Urine may leak out due to weakness of the bladder.

Reproductive Organs
- Giddiness and faintness before periods.
- Heavy, contracted sensations in womb with pains.
- Period pains extend into the back and down the thighs.

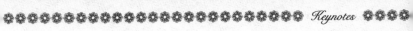

- Threatened miscarriage from anxiety or fear.
- Unproductive labour pains with very slow dilation of cervix, or 'backache' labour.

Sleep
- Wakes abruptly with a jerk from sleep.
- Fitful, disturbed sleep with general restlessness from aches and pains.

Worse from	*Better for*
Hot or overheated rooms	Moderate warmth
Humid weather	Fresh air
Cold draughts	Headaches are relieved by
Direct sunlight	passing large quantities of urine

Hepar sulph

Mental/Emotional Picture
- Terrific physical and mental sensitivity with frequent outbursts of irritability and bad temper.
- Quick to anger and generally difficult to get on with when ill.
- May be violent with temper and frustration.
- Hypersensitive to, and unable to stand any, physical pain or discomfort.

Fever
- Hypersensitive to cold draughts of air: has to be kept warm and snug or she feels terrible.
- Feels much worse for uncovering any part of the body.
- Perspires quickly and profusely after making the least physical effort.
- Perspiration often has a nasty, offensive odour.

Eyes
- Extreme sensitivity to light.
- Tendency to develop conjunctivitis or recurrent styes with sticky, yellow discharge.

Nose and Throat
- The slightest contact with cold air leads to immediate sneezing.
- Pain and inflammation of the sinuses with thick, yellow, nasty-smelling mucus.
- Pain and pressure at the root of the nose with sinus problems.
- Sore throat with sensation as though a fish bone or sharp object were sticking in sides of throat.
- Pains are often worse in the right side of the throat and may extend to the ear.
- Severely inflamed or septic tonsils with yellow-coloured ulcers.
- Laryngitis which feels much worse for exposure to cold.

Chest
- Severe coughing spasms which are made worse by slightest contact with cold air or uncovering.
- Rattling, productive cough with lots of mucus that is very difficult to dislodge.
- Feels sick and sweaty from the effort of bringing up phlegm.
- Throat and chest are better for warm drinks.

Digestion
- Severe belching with distension and swelling of stomach.
- Painless diarrhoea brought on immediately after eating.

Sleep
- Restless and sweaty at night and drowsy during the day.

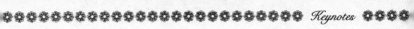

Skin

- Slow-healing skin with the smallest cut festering readily.
- Especially appropriate for boils and spots that are slow to come to a head, provided the general symptoms agree.
- Wounds and skin problems are extra sensitive to contact with cold air.

Worse from	*Better for*
Cold draughts	Warmth in any form
Cold food and drink	After eating
Light touch	Humid, warm weather
Lying on the painful area	
Morning and evening	

Hypericum

This remedy has a special affinity for injured areas that are rich in nerve supply, for example, crushed fingers or toes.

Mental/Emotional Picture

- Distress, sadness or drowsiness following an accident.

Head

- Headaches that follow a fall which involves the base of the spine.

General Features

- Crushing pains in fingers, toes or base of the spine after an accident.
- Damaged areas are extra-sensitive to touch.
- Injured parts are so sensitive that the slightest movement causes distress and weeping.
- Pain is especially strong on rising from sitting.
- Darting, intermittent pains shoot away from injured spot.

Worse from	Better for
Movement	Keeping absolutely still
Touch	
Damp, cold air	

Ignatia

One of the most likely remedies to be needed in situations of emotional stress, grief, and the shock of hearing bad news.

Mental/Emotional Picture
- Those who are in need of Ignatia are often in an excitable, nervous or extra-sensitive state.
- Very helpful in easing the symptoms of homesickness where there is an excessive amount of disorientation and distress.
- May be very upset, but bottle up emotions until they explode in hysterical trembling and crying.
- Contradictory moods: laughter alternates with tears, or anger with guilt and remorse.
- Hypersensitive to noise, criticism or pain.
- Feels misunderstood and resentful: may sigh all the time.

Head
- Headaches may follow stress, grief, shock or strong smells.
- Sharp pain as though a nail were sticking into the side or back of the head.

Nose and Throat
- Marked sensation of a lump in the throat which makes it very difficult to swallow.
- Persistent sore throat or loss of voice since emotional strain, trauma or upset.

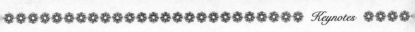

Digestion
- Lots of saliva in the mouth which tastes bitter.
- Hiccoughing and belching which are aggravated by eating.
- Spasmodic, cramping pains with constipation.
- Contradictory symptom of soft stools being harder to pass than hard ones.
- Diarrhoea without pain that is brought on by emotional stress.

Reproductive Organs
- Menstrual problems that are related to hormonal disturbances and imbalances.
- Colicky period pains which feel better lying down, applying pressure or from changing position.
- Dark, clotted, heavy, offensive flow.
- Often needed for post-natal problems such as depression or unpredictable mood swings.

Sleep
- Twitches, jerks and jolts in light sleep: wakes easily.
- Limbs jerk on going to sleep.
- Moans and whimpers in sleep.

Worse from
Emotional upset or shock
Bereavement
Fear or worry
Suppressing feelings
Yawning
Strong odours, such as
    tobacco smoke
Eating sugary foods
Pressure on non-painful areas
Exposure to cold

Better for
Being distracted
Warmth
Eating
Pressure to painful parts

Ipecac

Mental/Emotional Picture
- Very impatient, bad-tempered and dissatisfied.
- Becomes irritable from the least provocation.
- Over-sensitive to noise, especially loud music.

Fever
- Sudden onset of feverishness.
- Very chilly with sensitivity to the least draught of cold air.
- Shivering and trembling.
- Although feverish there is a lack of thirst.

Head
- Sick headache that involves the whole head.
- Terrible nausea with headache that makes the sufferer look terribly pale and ill.

Eyes
- Pains in the eyes with watering and sensitivity to light.

Nose and Throat
- Tendency to nosebleeds with blocked nostrils.
- Blood-stained mucus when nose runs.

Chest
- Coughing spasms come on suddenly with lots of rattling and wheezing in chest.
- Bouts of coughing cause gagging and often end in vomiting.
- Dry, irritating cough from tickling and irritation in air passages.
- Breathing problems make it difficult to lie flat: must sit up to catch breath.

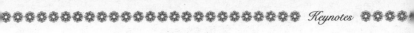

Digestion
- Awful, persistent nausea accompanies all symptoms.
- Sick feeling is not relieved by anything, including vomiting.
- Swollen, distended abdomen with constant desire to pass a stool.
- Greenish, watery diarrhoea.

Reproductive Organs
- Periods are irregular and very heavy: bleeding between periods.
- Tendency to haemorrhage with faintness and nausea.
- Flow is very flooding, gushing and bright red in colour.
- Terrible morning sickness in pregnancy which is made worse for the slightest movement.
- Excessively heavy bleeding during and after childbirth.

Worse from	*Better for*
Being overheated or too cold	Keeping as still as possible
Eating	Fresh air
The slightest movement	Firm pressure

Kali bich

Mental/Emotional Picture
- Lethargic and listless.
- Averse to anything that involves mental or physical effort.
- Anxiety about meeting new people.
- Poor memory with exhaustion.

Head

- Migraines with nausea and vomiting that are worse at night.
- Sinusitis with pains at the root of the nose.

Eyes

- Sensitive eyes that burn and itch.
- Recurrent conjunctivitis with heat and redness of the eyeball.
- Eyelids become red and swollen at the edges.

Ears

- Chronic ear pain with yellow, offensive-smelling discharge.

Nose and Throat

- Blocked nose from sticky, yellow discharge.
- Catarrah at back of throat which is stringy, stubborn and difficult to raise.
- Irritating sensation as though a hair is resting on the tongue.
- Sore throat with water-logged, enlarged uvula.
- Pains in throat are soothed by warm drinks.

Chest

- Feels as though there is a weight on chest on waking which is relieved on bringing up mucus.
- Cough is worse on waking in the morning and may be accompanied by back pain. It is relieved by lying down and by warmth.
- When coughing occurs after eating, food is vomited back up.

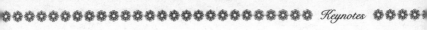

Digestion
- Headaches with stomach upsets that are worse from eating.
- Stomach feels more comfortable for belching.
- Anxiety and apprehension in the stomach.
- Persistent constipation with lethargy and headache.
- Involuntary passage of pale stools.

Kidneys and Bladder
- Constant urge to pass water during the day and night.
- Burning sensation during and after urinating.
- Fluid retention due to problems with kidney function.
- Low back discomfort or stitching pains.

Sleep
- Very drowsy and unrefreshed by sleep: wakes with a start around 2 a.m. from breathlessness, nausea, or feeling hot and sweaty.
- As a result of disturbed sleep feels exhausted during the day.
- Sleep is disturbed by upsetting dreams.

Worse from	*Better for*
Winter weather	Summer weather
Exposure to cold winds	Movement
Stooping	Warmth
Touch	Firm pressure
Waking from sleep	Being in bed
Feeling hungry	
Being alone	
Feeling too hot	
2–5 a.m.	

Kali carb

Mental/Emotional Picture

- Full of complaints and feels at odds with everyone and everything.
- Jumpy, nervous, and inclined to be over-sensitive to noise or shocks of any kind.
- Highly strung, irritable and edgy from over-tiredness.
- Lots of fears including a specific fear of being alone. Also afraid of the supernatural.
- Although dislikes being alone and seeks company, sympathy is rejected.

Head

- Burning pains in scalp or sinuses above eyes, or in cheek-bones.
- Pains are made much worse for contact with cold air and relieved by being wrapped-up warmly.

Eyes

- Eyelids are puffy with sharp pains in the eyes.

Nose and Throat

- Nose blocks up in a warm atmosphere which eases headache.
- Nasal passages feel uncomfortably dry and the nose looks generally very red, inflamed and swollen.
- Recurrent colds with loss of voice.
- Sticking, sharp pains in throat with a feeling of swallowing over a ball or lump in larynx.

Chest

- Chilly feeling in chest with wheezing and vomiting.
- Chronic, persistent, offensive-tasting catarrh may hang on from a previous illness that has not fully cleared up.

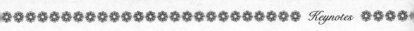

- Yellowish-green mucus that is lumpy and very difficult to raise.
- Dry, hacking cough with swollen upper eyelids.

Digestion
- Marked distension and swelling in abdomen that comes on after eating.
- Colicky pains that are eased by warmth, hot drinks, and hot-water bottles. Bends double with pains.
- Constipation or diarrhoea with burning sensations in rectum and anus.

Kidneys and Bladder
- Desire to pass water frequently with burning pains during and after urination.

Reproductive Organs
- Very chilly with cramping pains before the period starts.
- Constipation with period pains.
- Very heavy flow that may not respond to conventional medical measures.
- Tendency to miscarry when pregnant.
- Low back pain in pregnancy or 'backache labour'.

Sleep
- Wakes from sleep with horrible nightmares in the early hours and can't get back to sleep again.

Worse from	*Better for*
Change in weather	Warm, moist weather
Cold air or draughts	Leaning forward
Least physical contact with painful parts	During the day

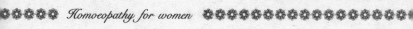

Lachesis

Mental/Emotional Picture

- Chatty and lively with a tendency to talk very quickly and constantly switch from one topic to another.
- Very mentally and physically sensitive with an aversion to being touched.
- Many problems stem from difficulties with sleep patterns: all symptoms are worse on waking from sleep.
- Works best at night and feels full of physical energy and bright ideas when it is time to go to bed.
- Fears falling asleep because of a conviction that she may die before waking.
- Starts and feels that she is falling as she is about to fall asleep.

Fever

- Volatile changes of temperature with constant fluctuations between heat and cold, or a constant disturbing sensation of waves or flushes of heat flowing through the body.
- Marked thirst for cool drinks and heavy perspiration.

Head

- Headaches or migraines characteristically come on when waking from sleep and usually affect the left side, or move from left to right.
- Bright light may trigger a headache or make an existing one much worse.
- Pains are eased by lying down, the onset of a nasal discharge, or warmth.

Eyes

- Painful, sensitive eyes that sting, itch and feel worse from being touched. Nevertheless, the instinct is to rub them constantly in search of relief.

Nose and Throat
- Sneezing with blocked nose in the morning.
- Nose feels more comfortable for the onset of a discharge, such as a nosebleed.
- Hoarseness on waking with tickling or sharp pain in throat.
- Irritation in throat provokes a choking sensation.
- All throat disorders are made worse by empty swallowing and feel better from swallowing solids. Cool drinks are generally soothing while warm things make discomfort worse.
- The throat is extra-sensitive to touch so that a polo-neck jumper or a scarf tied around the neck cause discomfort.
- Sore throats are often left-sided or begin on the left and move to the right.

Digestion
- Bloating and distention are relieved by passing a stool.
- Stools are difficult to pass because of throbbing pains in rectum or bleeding haemorrhoids.

Reproductive Organs
- Especially indicated for menopausal symptoms such as severe hot flushes, flooding periods with severe clotting, or violent mood swings.
- Severe PMS with left-sided ovarian pain, irritability to the point of frenzy, and such abrupt changes of mood that the sufferer becomes unrecognisable from herself when well.
- All of the above symptoms are relieved and improved as soon as the flow begins.

Sleep

- Terrible sleep problems including night sweats, feelings of panic and suffocation, anxiety and panic attacks. There is a general fear of going to sleep because all symptoms are worse on waking.
- Dreams may be horrific leading to confusion and disorientation on waking.

Skin

- Skin tends to flush easily with a tendency to broken capillaries, varicose veins, and a general blotchy, purple tinge. Boils or abscesses form readily with the affected area looking red or purple.

Worse from	*Better for*
Going to sleep	Fresh, open air
Heat	Cool drinks or cool applied locally
Overheated rooms	Onset of discharges
At night	Movement
Exposure to draughts	Eating
Heat of the sun	As the day goes on
Alcohol	
Feeling constricted	
Before a period	

Ledum

Mental/Emotional Picture

- Withdrawn, cross and irritable.

Fever

- Although feeling generally chilly, finds the warmth of the bed unbearable and flings off covers in an effort to cool down.
- Very thirsty for cold water.

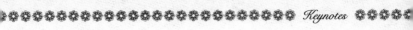

Head

- Pressing pains with headache that are relieved by fresh air and made worse by being covered.

General Features

- Pains are much worse from contact with warmth and better for cold applications or cool bathing.
- Pains move rapidly from site to site, and often tend to move in an upward direction.
- Whole body is bruised and aching.
- Swollen, hot joints that do not look red.
- Hard, painful swellings with tearing pains.

Skin

- Itchy eruptions are worse on covered parts of the body and react badly to the warmth of the bed, but feel immediately relieved by contact with cool air or water. Eruptions are crusty around the nose and mouth.

Worse from	Better for
Warmth in general	Cold in any form
At night	Contact with cool air
Being too warmly dressed	Bathing in cold water
Walking	Resting

Lycopodium

Mental/Emotional Picture

- Full of anxieties and insecurities: especially anxious anticipating an event that involves public speaking, such as delivering a speech or business presentation. Although lacking in confidence beforehand, when the event occurs, it goes very well.
- Dislikes too much attention and fussing, but also fears

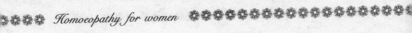

being totally alone: feels happiest in the knowledge that someone is within calling distance if needed.

- Specific fears of the dark, ghosts and strangers. Also very unhappy at feeling hemmed in or having constricting clothing around the neck or waist.
- Constantly preoccupied with worry over finances and fear of losing self-reliance. This is linked to the ultimate anxiety about fear of failure and losing control.
- Sensitive to pain, noise and music.
- Moves, speaks and eats very quickly. Words get jumbled up because of speaking so rapidly.
- Extremely sensitive to criticism and flies off the handle if corrected.
- Tendency to forgetfulness and confusion when overtired.

Fever
- Although chilly, dislikes being too warm or spending time in rooms that are stuffy or airless.
- Sudden flushes of heat.

Head
- Crushing, violent headaches that are made worse by warmth, becoming overheated and lying down.
- Headaches may be brought on by eating late.
- Pains are eased by cool, fresh air, and moving gently about.

Eyes
- Recurrent styes and other eye problems with very sticky, pussy discharges.

Nose and Throat
- Recurrent colds with sinus involvement and very blocked nasal passages.

- Thick, yellowy-green catarrh which settles at the back of the throat.
- Choking and burning sensations in the throat.
- Ulcerated throat which feels better for warm and worse for cold drinks.

Chest

- Persistent coughing causes a severe headache. Coughing bouts are brought on by breathing deeply or by swallowing saliva.

Digestion

- Stomach fills very quickly when eating: often begins a meal feeling hungry, but cannot eat very much without becoming overfull. Becomes hungry again within an hour or two of eating.
- Burning sensations in stomach come on immediately after eating and are relieved by warm drinks and aggravated by cold.
- Digestive problems often come on from 'nerves' or anticipatory anxiety before an exam or stressful event. This leads to lots of rumbling, gurgling, 'butterflies' in the stomach, and diarrhoea or very loose stools.
- Abdomen is so uncomfortable any pressure or constriction from a waistband or tight belt must be loosened.
- Accumulation of wind in the abdomen or production of excess acid in stomach leading to heartburn and indigestion.

Kidneys and Bladder

- Urine is cloudy, dark and strong-smelling or very pale.
- Aching pains in the sides before urinating which are relieved when urine has been passed.
- Urge to pass water very frequently at night.

Reproductive Organs
- Very severe period pains with cramps in the lower back and front of the thighs.
- Pains are relieved by drawing knees into the abdomen.
- Intense vaginal itching with, or without, fishy-smelling, copious discharge.
- Tendency to hot flushes and ready perspiration.

Skin
- Terrific irritability and dryness of the skin leading to violent itching and burning pains. These are much worse for becoming warm in bed and are soothed by contact with cool applications.
- Intense itching of the scalp with scaling of the scalp and dandruff.
- Hair is also dry and nails are brittle and break easily.

Worse from	*Better for*
The afternoons and early evening	Open air
	Uncovering
Warm, stuffy rooms or being overheated	Warm drinks
	Moderate warmth
Cold draughts	Loosening clothes
Touch	Gentle exercise
Weight of bedclothes	
Overtiredness	
On waking	

Mercurius

Mental/Emotional Picture
- Very anxious, fearful and restless for no obvious reason: finds it impossible to stay in one position for long.

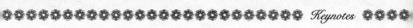

- All physical and mental symptoms are much worse at night.
- Either hurried and flustered or completely apathetic and indifferent.
- Depression with poor memory and distorted time sense.

Fever

- Very heavy, offensive-smelling perspiration that is worse at night.
- When perspiring extreme thirst is present.
- Hot flushes alternate with cold chills and shivering.

Head

- Head is sensitive all over, with head pains that are worse at night and on waking, and better from being up and about. The left side of the head may be more affected than the right.

Eyes

- Discomfort is made worse from heat and during the night.

Nose and Throat

- Sore, raw nostrils with offensive, green, thick discharge.
- It is difficult to swallow from dryness and soreness in the throat, but feels compelled to do so because of the increased amount of saliva.
- Persistent or frequently occurring swollen glands.

Chest

- Nauseating coughing spasms that are worse at night and from lying down.

Digestion
- Unpleasant, metallic, sweet taste with increased amount of saliva.
- Tongue feels and looks enlarged so that it takes the imprint of teeth around the edges.
- Cramping pains and diarrhoea are aggravated by bending forwards.
- Watery, burning diarrhoea gets more intense as night approaches.

Reproductive Organs
- Stinging, burning pains on ovulation.
- Terribly itchy vaginal discharge with maddening irritation which is worse at night and on passing urine.

Sleep
- Although drowsy by day, terrible insomnia occurs at night with overwhelming restlessness and physical unease. Sweating is especially marked at night and may have an offensive smell.

Worse from	Better for
Night and in the evening	Resting
In bed	Moderate temperatures
Extremes of heat or cold	
Draughts of cold air	
Perspiring	
Touch	
Lying on the right side	

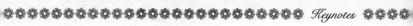

Natrum mur

Mental/Emotional Picture

- May experience contrary emotions, moving from one extreme mood to another.
- Rejects any form of physical affection or sympathy when upset, just wants to be left alone to get on with it.
- Intense dislike of being seen to cry: feels it is a sign of weakness, or something to be ashamed of.
- Averse to outward displays of emotion: keeps her emotions very guarded.
- Complaints often follow grief which has been unexpressed or not come to terms with.
- If upset, cries in private or may bottle up anger and resentment.
- All emotional and physical symptoms are much worse for hormonal changes, for example, at puberty, pre-menstrually, or at the menopause.

Head

- Headaches are associated with onset of periods, and may be much worse before, during or after a period.
- Head pains may also be brought on by delayed meal times: face may go pale with pain.
- Headache is worse for movement in general: pains are eased by lying down and sleeping it off.
- Becomes giddy and sick from travelling: may also develop a headache.

Eyes

- Eyes feel dry and gritty or water easily, especially if walking in strong, cold winds. Hay fever may also affect the eyes making them sensitive, itchy and swollen.

Nose and Throat

- Recurrent colds, rhinitis, or hay fever symptoms that start with bouts of repeated sneezing.
- Nasal discharge is copious and clear as though a hot tap has been turned on. This can alternate with very dry, uncomfortable obstruction of the nose.
- If it is running, nose pours clear discharge on bending forwards.
- Very runny nose alternates with dry, blocked feeling with nasal discharge that looks like egg white.
- Hoarse throat with irritated, tickling sensation.

Digestion

- Dry mouth and lips with characteristic crack in the middle of lips, or in the corners of the mouth.
- Recurrent cold sores that break out around the mouth and nose. These may be triggered by emotional stress, colds, or exposure to sunlight.
- Craving for or strong aversion to salty foods.
- Long-term constipation with severe straining to pass hard, dry stools.

Kidneys and Bladder

- Tendency to pass very large quantities of pale urine.
- Leakage of urine when walking, sneezing or coughing.
- General sense of lack of tone of pelvic organs including bladder.

Reproductive Organs

- Periods may be early and very heavy, or late with a scanty flow.
- Low back pains with or without actual prolapse of the womb. These are relieved by sitting or lying with firm pressure at the hollow of the back.

- Dryness of the vagina leads to an aversion to or lack of interest in intercourse because of the pain it causes.
- Fluid retention before periods leading to breast swelling and tenderness, and discomfort around the waist.

Skin
- Exposure to strong sunlight leads to hiving, 'prickly heat' and generally itchy, irritated, blotchy skin.
- Skin is badly affected by warmth when sensitive and feels more comfortable for cold compresses and exposure to open air.
- Dry quality to the skin with a tendency to crack easily, especially during the winter months.

Worse from	*Better for*
Emotional stress	Being alone
Sympathy and consolation	Open air
Overexcitement	Fasting
Crying in public	Gentle movement
After sleep	Cold bathing
Extreme temperatures	
Sunlight and hot weather	
Stuffy, overheated rooms	
Exercise	
Touch or pressure	

Nux vomica

This is one of the first remedies to consider in a 'hangover' situation or nausea following a general period of indulgence. It is also often indicated for symptoms following a course of conventional medication, such as constipation or general digestive upsets.

Mental/Emotional Picture
- Very touchy, irritable and easily provoked.
- Quickly frustrated and discontented.
- Sensitive on mental and physical levels with chronic sleeping problems.
- Reacts badly to being corrected or criticised, also does not respond well to sympathy or consolation.
- Because of demanding a lot of herself, someone who benefits from this remedy often resorts to stimulants, such as large quantities of caffeine, in order to keep going. She may also need regular quantities of alcohol in order to relax.
- Jittery and unable to switch off after work.
- Anxieties about health, work, the future and financial security.
- Very competitive and inclined to be a perfectionist.
- Because of her reliance on stimulants to keep going and sedatives to unwind, addiction may become an additional problem.

Fever
- Chilly and irritable when feverish with terrible dislike of the slightest draught of cold air. Although looking flushed and hot, she must be well covered.

Head
- Sick headaches with constipation and total lack of appetite.
- Headache feels better for warmth and firm pressure.
- Constricting head pains that are relieved by a cat nap.
- Classic tension headaches that stem from tightness at the back of the neck.

Eyes
- Burning, itching, smarting eyes.
- Severe sensitivity to light on waking with profuse watering and irritation of eyes.

Nose and Throat
- Lots of sneezing with raw feeling in throat
- Nose is either stuffed up and dry or runs like a tap.
- Pains in throat shoot to the ears periodically.
- Cold symptoms are generally more uncomfortable indoors and better in the fresh air.

Chest
- Very severe headaches accompany coughing bouts.
- Tickling, irritating dry cough that is worse at night.
- Coughing spasms are relieved by warm drinks and made worse by cold draughts of air.

Digestion
- Persistent nausea with severe difficulty in vomiting. However, once food is expelled from the stomach relief is felt straight away.
- Indigestion, wind and sharp pains that are made worse by eating or pressure and feel better for warmth.
- Stressful lifestyle and regular intake of convenience foods, strong tea, coffee and alcohol make stomach problems worse.
- Constipation with lots of straining and urging, but stool seems to slip back rather than being expelled.

Kidneys and Bladder
- Right-sided, burning kidney pain with terrible difficulty in urinating.
- Discomfort in bladder is particularly severe at night.
- Itching sensation when urinating.

Reproductive Organs
- Chilly and faint with period pains.
- Severe PMS with dreadful irritability and anger to the point of becoming violent.
- Morning sickness, persistent nausea and headaches in pregnancy.
- Distressing vomiting in labour with awful difficulty in bringing up stomach contents. Retching may be dry and painful.

Sleep
- Light, fitful sleep which is disturbed by frightening dreams.
- Wakes from light sleep feeling unrefreshed and anxious.
- Wakes in the early hours feeling fine but after falling asleep again feels tired and heavy-headed.
- Always feels better for a cat nap if tired during the day.
- May resort to sleeping pills in order to sleep.

Worse from	*Better for*
Cold in general, especially cold draughts of air	Warmth
	Resting
On waking	Undisturbed sleep
Disturbed or interrupted sleep	As the day goes on
	Humid weather
Eating	Passing a stool
Stimulants including strong coffee and caffeinated drinks	

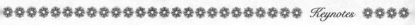

Phosphorus

Mental/Emotional Picture

- Easily exhausted on mental and physical levels.
- Anxious and full of fears: of thunder, being alone, illness, and of the dark.
- Craves reassurance and physical affection.
- Very sensitive and reactive to all sorts of stimuli: light, noise, colour, touch, music and perfume.
- May have a strongly developed sense of the psychic: sensitive to atmospheres and people.
- Very extrovert, vivacious and outgoing when feeling energetic.
- When exhausted becomes rapidly apathetic and totally indifferent.

Fever

- Subject to sudden variations and alternations in blood flow causing chilliness with sporadic flushes of heat.
- Although complaining of burning sensations, feet and legs may feel icy-cold.
- When feverish there may be an unquenchable thirst for ice-cold drinks which are vomited back as soon as they become warmed in the stomach.

Head

- Headache is made worse by warm, stuffy rooms and lying down.
- Pains are relieved by exposure to fresh, cool air and eating a little.
- Headache and weak, sickly feeling may be brought on by going too long between meals or from sensitivity to the atmospheric turbulence before a storm.
- Face is flushed with headache.

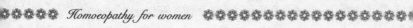

Nose and Throat

- Dry, blocked nostrils which make breathing difficult at night.
- Nasal discharge may be yellowy-green and unpleasant smelling.
- Colds go straight down to the throat and chest, often leading to swollen, inflamed glands in the neck.
- Throat is sensitive to touch and to cold air.
- Constant need to cough in order to clear the throat.
- Painless hoarseness or complete loss of voice.

Chest

- Irritating, dry cough that is worse for lying down and changing temperatures.
- Chest feels most comfortable when propped up in bed on a few pillows.
- Tight, wheezy chest that feels better for warmth.
- Yellow-coloured phlegm.

Digestion

- Burning stomach pains that are temporarily relieved by cold drinks.
- Warm drinks and food may lead to vomiting.
- Nausea and vomiting are much worse in an overheated, stuffy room.
- Very profuse, painless diarrhoea that may be passed involuntarily.
- Diarrhoea may come on during, or be made worse by, hot weather.

Reproductive Organs

- Tearful and very depressed with PMS.
- When period comes the flow is heavy and long lasting.

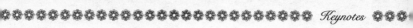

- Hot flushes, anxiety, palpitations, and flooding periods during the menopause.
- Bright red, clotted flow.
- May be needed before, or during labour where panic and anxiety are causing a lot of distress.

Worse from	*Better for*
Early evening	Reassurance
Darkness	Uninterrupted sleep
Being alone	Warmth
Overexcitement	Eating regularly
Thunderstorms	Being massaged or given
Lying on the left side	physical affection and
	comfort

Pulsatilla

Mental/Emotional Picture
- Changeable, shifting moods moving from weepiness to irritability or happiness very quickly.
- May be anxious and in need of reassurance and consolation.
- Reacts well to sympathy, company and physical displays of affection.
- If unhappy feels much better after a good cry in sympathetic company.
- Timid and in need of a lot of attention.
- Emotional symptoms and insecurities are particularly marked before a period or when pregnant.
- May become very depressed if she feels ignored, uncared for, or unsupported.
- Fears crowds, open spaces, being alone, and losing her reason.

Fever

- Very chilly with a strong dislike of becoming overly warm in a stuffy room. Although the mouth is often dry and parched with fever, there is no thirst.
- Hot and cold flushes alternate with a dislike of being too well-covered in bed.

Head

- Headache with upset stomach from eating too rich a diet or very fatty foods.
- Pains are worse after eating or come on during the evening.
- Headaches feel better from firm pressure or a cool flannel. Gentle movement out of doors in the fresh air also helps.

Eyes

- Conjunctivitis with yellow, thick discharge that sticks the lids together overnight.
- Itchy, burning eyes with a constant desire to rub them.
- Frequent styes that affect the lower lid.

Nose and Throat

- The nose feels sore and swollen during a cold.
- Blocked feeling alternates from side to side. It improves in fresh air and gets worse indoors (especially if the room is overheated or stuffy).
- Loss of taste and smell with a heavy cold.
- Constant catarrh which is yellowy-green, thick and bland.
- Dry, sore throat with no thirst.

Chest

- Dry cough on waking which develops into a loose and more productive cough at night.
- Uncomfortable feeling in chest on lying down which is relieved by sitting up or moving about.
- Yellowy-green phlegm.

Digestion

- Tongue is heavily coated and coloured white or yellow.
- Nasty taste in dry mouth with no thirst.
- Vomiting may follow overexcitement, emotional upset or stress.
- Chilly sensation with persistent nausea that feels worse in a stuffy or overheated room.
- Burning indigestion is made worse by warm food or drink and better for cool.
- Violent, burning diarrhoea that is worse at night and may be triggered by eating too much fruit or ice-cream.

Kidneys and Bladder

- Easy leaking of urine especially when sitting, walking, coughing or lying down.
- Recurrent cystitis with burning and smarting that is much worse for contact with warmth and better for cool.
- Pain and discomfort persists even after passing water.
- Bladder symptoms are worse when lying on the back.

Reproductive Organs

- Late onset of periods with a tendency for irregularity: never knows when the next one might be due.
- The flow may be changeable, being heavy or clotted and then changing to a very scanty flow.
- Severe symptoms of PMS with tender swollen breasts and extreme mood swings. Predominant emotion is often weepiness.
- Recurrent problems with thrush which causes violent itching and a thick, whitish-yellow discharge.
- Menopausal symptoms include abrupt temperature changes with intolerance of heat, stress incontinence, low back pain with prolapse, and very irregular, flooding periods.

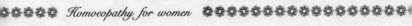

- This remedy is often needed in pregnancy where vomiting lasts all day, or gets worse during the evening or at night.
- Varicose veins, thrush or cystitis may be especially troublesome in pregnancy.
- During labour pains are feeble, changeable, or unproductive.

Sleep
- Sleepy on going to bed but wakes from becoming overheated or too sweaty during the night.
- Throws off bedclothes, gets too chilly, then pulls them back on again. As a result, can't get comfortable and feels constantly restless.
- Often sleeps with arms extended above the head and feet pushed out of the covers in search of a cool spot.

Skin
- Terrible itching which is made worse by contact with heat in any form. Discomfort is eased by contact with cool air and washing in cool water.

Worse from	*Better for*
Stuffy rooms	Cool food or drink, washing, and cool applied locally
Heat	
Heavy clothing or bedclothes	Fresh, cool, open air
Humidity	Gentle exercise
Resting	Sympathy and attention
Lying down	Physical displays of affection
Evening and at night	A good cry in sympathetic company
Pregnancy	
	Firm pressure to painful area

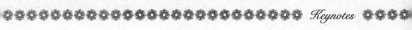

Rhus tox

This is a remedy that is most often indicated for aches and pains which are much better for keeping on the move, and worse for resting, or exposure to cold and damp. A great deal of stiffness and sharp, shooting pains accompany joint and muscle problems.

Mental/Emotional Picture
- Extreme degree of mental and physical restlessness which is especially strong at night.
- Withdrawn, depressed, apathetic and can't be bothered with anything.
- Anxiety, sadness and weepiness over things that wouldn't normally cause an upset.
- Fears are worse at night when lying in bed.
- Bursts into tears for no obvious reason.

Fever
- Delirium when feverish: may mutter in disturbed sleep.
- Unquenchable thirst for cold drinks, especially at night.
- Sweaty and trembling with high temperature which is aggravated by warm drinks.

Head
- Severe headache that is eased by warmth and bending the head backwards.
- Headache may follow anger or frustration.

Eyes
- Stiff feeling in eyeballs with very watery, irritated eyes.
- Styes with stiff sensation in eyelids.

Nose and Throat
- Sneezing and frequent nosebleeds on waking.

- Hoarseness on speaking which improves the more the voice is used.

Chest
- Dry, tickly cough that is brought on by exposure to the least draught of cold, damp air.
- Coughing leads to severe headache.
- Raw feeling in air passages with unpleasant bloody or salty taste in mouth.

Digestion
- Dry, sore cracked lips and mouth with recurrent cold sores.
- Inflamed, sore tongue with red triangular tip.
- Severe stomach pains are relieved by gentle motion and bending double.
- Severe, painless morning diarrhoea.
- Exhausted with diarrhoea which may be passed involuntarily.

Sleep
- Very fitful, restless sleep, especially after midnight.
- Feels exhausted on waking from unrefreshing sleep and disturbed dreams.
- Constantly moves about the bed in search of a comfortable position.

Skin
- Skin feels constantly irritated in bed at night with permanent desire to scratch. Puffy skin eruptions itch and burn intolerably.

Worse from	*Better for*
Damp, cold weather	Warmth
Resting	Continued movement,
Lying still	provided it doesn't exhaust

Standing
Initial movement
After midnight
Scratching

Warm bathing
Heat applied locally
Wrapping up warmly
Warm, dry weather

Sepia

Mental/Emotional Picture

- Very depressed, down, and bad-tempered.
- Although weepy, having a good cry does little to relieve feelings of depression.
- Terribly irritable and impatient with family.
- Indifferent to partner and averse to any sexual contact.
- Totally lacking in energy and drive: feels droopy and dragged down.

  Often indicated for depressive feelings during the menopause, after childbirth, or during severe PMS if other guiding symptoms fit.
- Feels mentally and emotionally improved after vigorous exercise, such as an aerobics class or a brisk walk.

Head

Giddiness on waking with poor circulation or low blood pressure.

Severe headaches which are one-sided with throbbing, shooting pains.

Migraines or headaches are made worse by light, noise and the atmosphere before a storm.

Taking exercise often eases the pain.

Terrible nausea with headache that is made much worse by strong odours, like cooking smells.

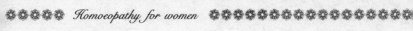

Eye
- Gritty sensation in the eyes with or without burning and watering.
- Visual disturbance such as zig-zags or sparks before the eyes.
- Temporary loss of vision or visual distortion may occur before a migraine.

Nose and Throat
- Frequent colds with dry, sore, crusty nostrils.
- Tip of the nose becomes inflamed and swollen.

Chest
- Troublesome, hacking cough that is worse on waking, or during the night.
- Coughing bouts lead to nausea, vomiting and retching.
- Pains and uneasiness in the chest feel better for pressing hands on the affected area.

Digestion
- Faintness and nausea come on for no apparent reason, or from missing regular meals.
- Eating can temporarily help nausea if it is caused by low blood sugar levels.
- Acidic pains, or a feeling of constant movement in the stomach.
- Constipation with small, dry, hard stools which are slow and difficult to pass.
- Even after a stool has been passed, a sense of fullness still remains in the rectum.
- Lots of pains after passing a stool from bleeding, inflamed haemorrhoids.

Kidneys and Bladder
- Strong sense of pressure in the bladder with constant

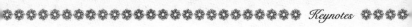

feeling of wanting to pass water, day and night.
- Strong-smelling, brightly coloured urine with possible reddish sediment.

Reproductive Organs
- Weariness and complete exhaustion before a period is due.
- Terrible PMS with mood swings, lethargy, irritability and delayed, scanty periods.
- Morning sickness that is much worse for going without food and better for a snack.
- Tendency to prolapse of the womb with a feeling as though everything was about to fall out.
- Symptoms are worse for standing or walking, and feel better for sitting cross-legged.
- Dryness of vagina during and after the menopause causes great distress and aversion to intercourse.
- Other menopausal symptoms include violent hot flushes with heavy sweating after a little physical effort.
- Itching in vagina with yellowy-green discharge.

Sleep
- Although drowsy during the day, unable to sleep at night.
- Stays awake for hours and feels totally unrefreshed on waking.
- Sweats and flushes may also be especially severe at night.

Skin
- Acne may develop at puberty, and eczema during the menopause.
- Urticaria (hiving) may be related to hormonal shifts, such as during ovulation or before a period.
- Itchy skin feels worse out of doors and better in a warm room. However, it is made worse by the heat of the bed.

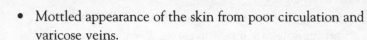

- Mottled appearance of the skin from poor circulation and varicose veins.

Worse from	*Better for*
Before, during or after a period	Vigorous activity, such as running, walking or dancing
Skipping meals	
Damp	Eating
Resting	Warmth
Perspiring	After sleep
Touch	Firm pressure
Mental effort	
Emotional demands	

Silica

Mental/Emotional Picture

- Full of anxiety, lack of confidence and insecurity about her ability to achieve anything.
- When undertaking anything, feels she is bound to fail.
- Phobia or obsessions about pointed objects such as pins or needles: may be terrified of injections.
- Develops fixed, rigid ideas that are very difficult to shift.
- Mental fatigue and lack of confidence leads to difficulty in making decisions.
- Becomes nervous and overwrought to the point of jumping and flinching at the slightest noise.
- Irritable and short-tempered from insecurity and lack of confidence.

Head

- Flushes of blood to the head which especially affect the crown and the right side.

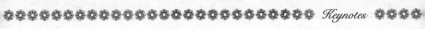

- Severe, bursting, recurrent headaches that start at the base of the skull and spread over the whole head.
- Tight pressure, heat, and wrapping-up warmly relieve head pains.
- Headaches are aggravated by exposure to cold, movement, light, and noise.

Eyes

- Dry, gritty sensations in eyes with watering in the open air.
- Visual disturbance and dizziness with headaches.

Nose and Throat

- Sneezing with alternately dry and running nose.
- Nasal passages may be uncomfortably blocked with painful sinuses.
- Persistent sore throats or tonsilitis with swollen glands.
- Salivary glands may also be very swollen and tender.

Chest

- Hoarseness with dry cough that is worse from cold drinks or talking.
- Irritating tickle in chest and cough may be relieved by warm drinks.
- A bad coughing fit leaves the sufferer exhausted and gasping.

Digestion

- Nausea with aversion to water, which tastes unpleasant, and warm food or drinks.
- Warmth is also soothing to abdominal pains and tenderness.
- Severe constipation with extreme difficulty in passing even soft stools.

- Anal fissure may be present, or terribly sensitive haemorrhoids.
- Sticking pains for some time after passing a stool.

Skin

- Skin tends to become infected very easily: even the smallest scratch quickly becomes septic and inflamed.
- Abscesses, boils and carbuncles recur, with very slow healing capacity.
- Scars from skin problems remain for a very long time.
- Bones may also be of very poor quality with a tendency to break easily.

Worse from	Better for
Exposure to cold air	Hot compresses
Cold weather	Being wrapped-up warmly
Pressure	Summer weather
Lying on painful part	
During periods	

Staphysagria

Mental/Emotional Picture

- Extremely angry and resentful, but smoulders and broods rather than spontaneously expressing emotions.
- Problems arise from an inability to express feelings of anger, humiliation, grief or rejection.
- Often indicated for situations of emotional and sexual abuse.
- Dwells on past events, suffering in silence about unfair treatment or injustices.
- Trembles and shakes with the force of suppressed anger.
- Insomnia from persistent frustrating thoughts.

- Depressed and apathetic leading to terrible problems with sleep pattern.
- Irritated and upset by slightest criticism.

Head
- Dizziness that is relieved by moving around and worse for lying down or sitting.
- Pains are mainly in the forehead, but the whole head may feel tight or numb.

Eyes
- Itchy margins of eyelids with tendency for styes to develop.

Digestion
- Irritation and discomfort in the stomach which is aggravated by smoking.
- Burning and pressure in the stomach with retching.
- Stomach pains are brought on by drinking cold water or getting very tense and irritable.
- Terribly sensitive haemorrhoids which sting and burn.

Kidneys and Bladder
- Constant need to pass water with burning that persists afterwards.
- Urine is very concentrated and dark-coloured.
- Cystitis may be brought on by intercourse: 'honeymoon cystitis'.

Reproductive Organs
- Increased libido or aversion to sexual contact with extra-sensitive, itchy vagina.
- Well indicated for depression or suppressed anger following a Caesarian delivery, episiotomy, hysterectomy, or any surgical procedure associated with feelings of

assault, violation or bitter disappointment (as in a difficult birth).

Skin
- Scaly or weepy eruptions which burn before and after scratching.
- Once one area has been scratched, itching moves to another place leading to an itch/scratch/itch cycle.
- Slow-healing wounds with persistent stinging pains.
- Sharp, stinging pains during and after shingles.

Worse from	*Better for*
Suppressed feelings	Warmth
Slight touch	Resting
Sexual activity	Uninterrupted sleep
Smoking	After breakfast
Early morning	
Mental effort	

Sulphur

Although frequently indicated for symptoms involving irritation and itching of the skin, because of its very dynamic and deep-acting nature, this remedy should be used very sparingly and with caution. Do not repeat it frequently over an extended period of time, especially where there is a history of skin problems, such as eczema or psoriasis.

Mental/Emotional Picture
- Lacks grit or staying power with regard to things that call for long-term stamina or persistence.
- Very irritable, touchy and sorry for herself.
- Impatient, short-tempered with a tendency to sulk when offended.

- Philosophical and wordy: tends to beat around the bush rather than saying what she means.
- Introspective and self-absorbed.
- Combination of fastidiousness with untidiness: study is chaotic while work that is produced is immaculate.
- Anxious, weepy and depressed during periods and the menopause.
- Strong aversion to washing because it always aggravates symptoms.

Fever

- Although very hot and flushed, overheated and draughty rooms are both disliked.
- Head is often uncomfortably hot while the feet are chilly, or feet may feel burning hot.
- Very thirsty for lots of cold drinks, but sweat is absent.

Head

- Weekend headaches are common.
- Headaches are worse out of doors or when stooping, and better for resting in a moderate temperature.

Eyes

- Redness around lid margins with a yellowish discharge that dries into crusts.
- Itching, redness and burning of the eyes.

Nose and Throat

- Nose is stuffed up when indoors and runs when outside.
- Frequent colds with thick, offensive, persistent nasal discharge.
- Discomfort in throat like a sensation of a ball or lump that won't move on swallowing.

Chest
- Pressure and tightness in chest that is worse at night.
- Must have windows open for fresh air.

Digestion
- Strong dislike of fat, eggs and milk.
- Ravenous appetite, especially around mid-morning.
- Queasy sensation in the stomach is much worse for skipping meals.
- Craving for spicy, fatty foods and alcohol which aggravate indigestion.
- Painless, early morning diarrhoea: has to rush to the toilet to get there in time.
- Alternation of constipation and diarrhoea.
- Red, sore, burning anus with diarrhoea.

Kidneys and Bladder
- Burning and smarting on passing water.
- Recurrent kidney problems with shivering, cold sweat and muscle aches on urinating.

Reproductive Organs
- Irregular periods with unpredictable flow.
- Hot flushes and shivering during the menopause with faint feelings.
- Prolapse of womb with bearing down sensations which are made much worse by standing.
- Itching and burning in vagina which may be much worse during the menopause.

Sleep
- Wakes regularly around 3 a.m. and can't get back to sleep. Violent starting on the verge of falling asleep.
- Always feels the need of more sleep: wants to lie in.

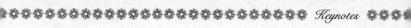

Skin

- Itchy, inflamed, unhealthy skin that burns after scratching.
- Itching is so intense that scratching leads to bleeding and weeping.
- Skin feels much worse for contact with heat in any form, such as warmth of the bed or bathing in warm water. May also be very sensitive to contact with wool.

Worse from
Heat and warmth
Getting warm in bed
Bathing
Eating
Waking
Mid-morning

Better for
Moderate temperatures
Lying on the right side

HOMOEOPATHIC REMEDIES AND THEIR ABBREVIATIONS

Remedy	Abbreviated name
Aconitum napelus	Aconite
Allium cepa	
Antimonium crudum	Ant crud
Antimonium tartaricum	Ant tart
Apis mellifica	Apis
Arnica montana	Arnica
Arsenicum album	Arsenicum alb
Belladonna	
Bryonia alba	Bryonia
Calcarea carbonica	Calc carb
Calcarea phosphorica	Calc phos
Calendula officinalis	Calendula
Cantharis	
Carbo vegetablilis	Carbo veg
Caulophyllum	Caul
Chamomilla	
Cimicifuga	Cimic
Colocythis	
Cuprum metallicum	Cuprum

Eupatorium perfoliatum	Eupatorium
Euphrasia	
Ferrum metallicum	Ferrum met
Ferrum phosphoricum	Ferrum phos
Gelsemium sempervirens	Gelsemium
Hepar sulphuris calcareum	Hepar sulph
Hypericum perfoliatum	Hypericum
Ignatia amara	Ignatia
Ipecacuana	Ipecac
Kali bichromium	Kali bich
Kali carbonicum	Kali carb
Kali muriaticum	Kali mur
Kreosotum	
Lachesis	
Ledum palustre	Ledum
Lycopodium	
Magnesia phosphorica	Mag phos
Mercurius solubilis	Mercurius
Natrum muriaticum	Nat mur
Nux vomica	
Phosphorus	
Phytolacca decandra	Phytolacca
Podophyllum	
Pulsatilla nigricans	Pulsatilla
Pyrogenium	Pyrogen
Rhus toxicodendron	Rhus tox
Rumex crispus	Rumex
Ruta graveolens	Ruta
Sanguinaria	
Silica	
Spongia tosta	Spongia

Sulphur
Symphytum officinale   Symphytum
Thuja occidentalis   Thuja
Urtica urens   Urtica
Veratrum album   Veratrum alb

FURTHER READING

*Homoeopathy for Mother and Baby: Pregnancy, birth, and the post-
natal year*, Miranda Castro, Macmillan, 1992
Homoeopathy for Women, Rima Handley, Thorsons, 1993
*The Woman's Guide to Homoeopathy: The Natural Way to a Healthier
Life for Women*, Dr Andrew Lockie and Dr Nicola Geddes,
Hamish Hamilton, 1992
Homoeopathic Medicines for Pregnancy and Childbirth, Dr Richard
Moskowitz, North Atlantic Books, 1992
*Natural Medicine for Women: Drug-free healthcare for women of all
ages*, Julian and Susan Scott, Gaia, 1991
*Every Woman's Lifeguide: How to achieve and maintain fitness, health
and happiness in today's world*, Dr Miriam Stoppard, Optima,
1988
Everywoman: A Gynaecological Guide for Life, Derek Llewellyn-
Jones, Penguin, 1993
The Well Woman's Self-Help Directory, Nikki Bradford, Sidgwick
and Jackson, 1990
The New Our Bodies Ourselves: A Health Book for and by Women,
Angela Phillips and Jill Rakusen, Penguin, 1989
*Hormone Replacement Therapy: Your Guide to Making an Informed
Choice*, Rosemary Nicol, Vermillion, 1993
Everything You Need to Know about Osteoporosis, Rosemary Nicol,
Sheldon Press, 1990
'HRT The Myths Exploded', Fiona Bawdon, *What Doctors Don't
Tell You*, 4: 9 (1994)

General books on homoeopathy

*The Complete Homoeopathy Handbook: A Guide to Everyday Health
Care*, Miranda Castro, Macmillan, 1990
*Everybody's Guide to Homoeopathic Medicines: Taking Care of
Yourself and Your Family with Safe and Effective Remedies*, Dr
Stephen Cummings and Dana Ullman, Gollancz, 1986

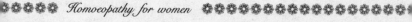

The Family Guide to Homoeopathy: The Safe Form of Medicine for the Future, Dr Andrew Lockie, Elm Tree Books, 1989

How to Use Homoeopathy, Dr Christopher Hammond, Element, 1991

Homoeopathic Medicine at Home, Maesimund Panos and Jane Heimlich, Corgi, 1980

Homoeopathy, Medicine for the 21st Century, Dana Ullman, Thorsons, 1989

Homoeopathy, Medicine for the New Man, George Vithoulkas, Thorsons, 1985

The Complete Book of Homoeopathy, Michael Weiner and Kathleen Goss, Bantam, 1982

Homoeopathy: Headway Lifeguides, Beth MacEoin, Headway, 1992

Homoeopathy for Babies and Children, Beth MacEoin, Headway, 1994

USEFUL ADDRESSES

Council for Complementary and Alternative Medicine
179 Gloucester Place
London NW1 6DX
Tel: 071 724 9103

Natural Medicines Society
Market Chambers
13A Market Place
Heanor
Derbyshire DE75 7AA
Tel: 0773 710002

British Complementary Medical Association
St Charles' Hospital
Exmoor Street
London W10 6DZ
Tel: 081 964 1206

The Society of Homoeopaths
2 Artizan Road
Northampton
NN1 4HU
Tel: 0604 21400

The British Homoeopathic Association
27a Devonshire Street
London WC1N 3HZ
Tel: 071 935 2163

The Homoeopathic Society
Hahnemann House
Powis Place
Great Ormond Street
London WC1N 1RJ

Ainsworths Homoeopathic Pharmacy
38 New Cavendish Street
London
W1M 7LH
Tel: 071 935 5330 (Daytime)
071 487 5252 (24 hour answering machine service)

Helios Homoeopathic Pharmacy
97 Camden Road
Tunbridge Wells
Kent TN1 2QP
Tel: 0892 536393

The Homoeopathic Supply Company
4 Nelson Road
Sherringham
Norfolk
NR26 8BU
Tel: 0263 824683

INDEX